DATE DUE

WITHDRAWN

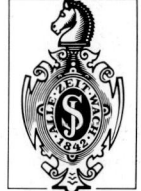

J. M. Connor

Soft Tissue Ossification

Foreword by Victor A. McKusick, MD

With 50 Figures

Springer-Verlag
Berlin Heidelberg New York Tokyo
1983

J.M. Connor, BSc, MB, ChB, MD, MRCP
Consultant in Medical Genetics
Duncan Guthrie Institute of Medical Genetics
Yorkhill, Glasgow G3 8SJ, Scotland

ISBN 3-540-12530-2 Springer-Verlag Berlin Heidelberg New York Tokyo
ISBN 0-387-12530-2 Springer-Verlag New York Heidelberg Berlin Tokyo

Library of Congress Cataloging in Publication Data
Connor, J.M. (James Michael), 1951– Soft tissue ossification.
Bibliography: p. Includes index. 1. Metaplastic ossification. I. Title. [DNLM: 1. Ossification, Pathologic. 2. Soft tissue neoplasms. 3. Myositis ossificans. QZ 180 C752s]
RC931.M47C65 1983 611'.018 83-10275
ISBN 0-387-12530-2 (U.S.)

This work is subject to copyright. All rights are reserved, whether the whole or part of the material is concerned, specifically those of translation, reprinting, re-use of illustrations, broadcasting, reproduction by photocopying, machine or similar means, and storage in data banks. Under §54 of the German Copyright Law where copies are made for other than private use, a fee is payable to 'Verwertungsgesellschaft Wort', Munich.

© by Springer-Verlag Berlin Heidelberg 1983
Printed in Great Britain

The use of registered names, trademarks, etc. in the publication does not imply, even in the absence of a specific statement, that such are exempt from the relevant protective laws and regulations and therefore free for general use.

Typeset by Wilmaset, Birkenhead, Merseyside
Printed by The Alden Press, Oxford

2128/3916-543210

To Mona and Rachel

Foreword

There is much good clinical medicine and much good biology, including genetics, in this monograph by Connor. His interest in soft tissue ossification was an outgrowth of his work on fibrodysplasia ossificans progressiva (FOP). Although FOP is a rarity, like other genetic diseases it has many implications for common problems of medical and surgical practice. The major problem of soft tissue ossification after total hip replacement (p. 27) is a case in point, as is also the ossification after severe burns (p. 31) and in paraplegics (p. 75).

FOP is a rare mutant state inherited as an autosomal dominant. Virtually all cases are the consequence of new mutation; the disorder goes no further in the family line because the affected persons rarely reproduce. Connor did a model job of ascertaining as completely as possible cases of FOP in England, and of studying a majority of them personally. This gave him a chance to estimate incidence and mutation rate, and to examine the effect of father's age on the occurrence of this disorder, as well as to provide a valid description of the range in variety of clinical manifestations and the natural history in an unbiased series.

In connection with all the disorders Connor discusses, not only FOP, a strong genetical theme is discernible. For example, the author points out that patients who would get ossification after surgical replacement of one hip are likely to suffer the same complication on the other side as well (p. 28). Post-burn soft tissue ossification of similar distribution has been noted in twins, neither of whom was seriously burned (p. 32). A patient has been reported with ossification in three separate primary neoplasms (p. 46). Brothers both developed ossification in upper midline abdominal surgical scars (p. 95). Osteoma cutis, an exceedingly rare disorder, has been described in mother and son (p. 101). Ossification of the posterior longitudinal ligament of the cervical spine (p. 91) is strikingly more frequent in Japanese than in other ethnic groups. Although a commonality in methods of medical and surgical management and lifestyle, and in other nongenetic 'risk factors', may explain in part these observations, they point nonetheless toward possible innate predisposition.

Here the reader will find fascinating bits of lore. What is the origin of the expression 'Charley horse'? (See p. 19.) How is traumatic ossification in the left deltoid muscle of American sailors related to a practice adopted from British naval tradition? (See p. 23.) What is the typical tendon ossification of the super-high divers of Acapulco? (See p. 27.) And, of course, from an earlier age there are the well-known 'cobbler's bone,' 'rider's bone' of the horseman, and 'drill bone' of the infantryman. Did Lot's wife who turned to a pillar of stone and the ancient Greeks who turned into stone after looking into the face of one of the Gorgon sisters have FOP? (See p. 54.)

A leading actor in this piece is the inducible osteogenic precursor cell (IOPC). Its regulation may be awry on a genetic basis in fibrodysplasia ossificans progressiva, and it probably represents the common pathogenetic pathway for much soft tissue ossification of an acquired nature. The biology and pathology of this cell will continue to be of great interest for some time to come, I suspect.

I can recommend this monograph enthusiastically to orthopedic surgeons, rheumatologists, radiologists, and sports physicians as well as to those who specialize in physical medicine and rehabilitation—indeed to all physicians who encounter the problem of soft tissue calcification and ossification.

Baltimore, Maryland
March 1983

Victor A. McKusick, MD

Preface

Bone is normally confined to the skeleton, where it has important mechanical and metabolic functions. In several diseases bone may also form in the soft tissues and result in physical disability. These diseases, although individually uncommon, collectively pose important clinical problems with regard to differential diagnosis and management.

Although such diseases are usually considered an orthopedic problem, patients not infrequently present to other specialists, notably rheumatologists, sports physicians and those concerned with rehabilitation medicine. In the subsequent differential diagnosis, collaboration between clinician, radiologist and pathologist is essential as diagnosis on the basis of clinical, radiological or pathological findings alone can be misleading. In this group of diseases correct diagnosis is crucial, since they differ widely in prognosis and therapy which is appropriate for one may be frankly harmful in another.

Soft tissue ossification receives consideration in all major textbooks of orthopedics, radiology and pathology. However, these accounts often fail to encompass current understanding of this group of diseases. Moreover, there appears to be a need for a monograph which combines these different standpoints for, as emphasized earlier, a collaborative approach to diagnosis is desirable.

This monograph was written with this approach in mind and is directed to the specialists who are involved in the day-to-day care of patients with ossifying lesions. Thus, its order follows the logical clinical approach. Chapter 1 deals with the differential diagnosis and Chapters 2 to 6 can then be consulted for a self-contained account of each disease which includes both medical and surgical aspects of management. In addition to outlining established facts, these chapters also indicate important areas of controversy.

The last three chapters serve both as an outline of the current status of research into the regulation of osteogenesis and to indicate the clinical implications of recent advances in this area. In a book of this size it is not possible to describe in detail all of the diseases in which amorphous calcification, as opposed to ossification, of the soft tissues can occur. Further, visceral calcification and ossification is given only brief mention.

Many people have influenced the preparation of this manuscript and

I am particularly grateful to: Prof. V.A. McKusick and Prof. E.A. Murphy (Departments of Medicine and Medical Genetics, The Johns Hopkins Hospital); Prof. D.A. Price Evans (Department of Medicine, University of Liverpool); Prof. Peter Beighton (Department of Human Genetics, University of Cape Town); Dr. Roger Smith, and Dr. Jim Triffitt (Nuffield Orthopaedic Centre, Oxford); and the specialists on both sides of the Atlantic who have allowed me to study their patients with soft tissue ossification.

I would also like to thank the University of Liverpool and the National Institute of Health (grant number T32 GM07471-05) for funding during my research on this group of diseases and during the preparation of this manuscript.

Baltimore, 1983   J.M. Connor

Contents

1 Differential Diagnosis of Soft Tissue Calcification 1

History 3
Physical Examination 6
Laboratory Tests 9
Radiology 9
Biopsy 14
Summary 14

2 Ossification After Major Trauma 17

Ossification After Repeated Minor Trauma 23
Hematoma Ossification 24
Post-traumatic Ossification of Ligaments and Tendons 25
Ossification After Hip Replacement 27
Ossification After Burns 31
Ossification After Tetanus 33

3 Tumor Ossification 38

Parosteal Osteosarcoma 38
Soft Tissue Osteosarcoma 40
Other Ossifying Connective Tissue Tumors 42
Ossifying Skin Tumors 43
Visceral Tumor Ossification 44
Pseudomalignant Myositis Ossificans 46

4 Fibrodysplasia Ossificans Progressiva 54

Prevalence 55
Clinical Features 55
Radiology 61
Laboratory Studies 65

Pathology	65
Etiology	67
Natural History	69
Management	70

5 Ossification in Neurological Conditions ... 75

History and Nomenclature	75
Prevalence	75
Clinical Features	77
Radiology	79
Pathology	80
Pathogenesis	81
Natural History	82
Management	82

6 Other Causes of Soft Tissue Ossification ... 87

Ossification in the Arthropathies	87
Ossification of the Posterior Longitudinal Ligament (OPLL)	91
Bridging of Lumbar Transverse Processes	92
Ossification in Surgical Incisions	93
Ossification in Chronic Venous Insufficiency	96
Hypoparathyroidism	98
Hereditary Hypophosphatemia	100
Primary Osteoma Cutis	101
Para-articular Ossification in Melorheostosis	102
Miscellaneous Causes	103

7 Experimental Production of Ectopic Bone ... 108

Traumatic Induction of Bone	108
Cellular Induction of Bone	109
Chemical Induction of Bone	110
Cells with Osteogenic Potential	112

8 Regulation of Osteogenesis ... 117

Origins of Osteogenic Cells	117
Normal Osteogenesis	118
Hormones and Osteogenesis	119
Alkaline Phosphatase and Osteogenesis	120
Vitamins and Osteogenesis	121
Trace Elements and Osteogenesis	122
Mechanical Stress and Osteogenesis	123
Electricity and Osteogenesis	124

Genes and Osteogenesis 124
Cellular Interactions and Osteogenesis 125
Medications and Osteogenesis 126
Other Influences on Osteogenesis 127

9 Conclusions and Clinical Implications 132

Subject Index 141

1 Differential Diagnosis of Soft Tissue Calcification

Deposition of calcium salts is normally restricted to the skeleton. Ectopic or heterotopic calcification refers to calcium deposition in any other tissue, and these may be subdivided into the soft tissues and the viscera. The soft tissues include: skin, fat, skeletal muscle, cartilage, fibrous connective tissue, blood vessels, peripheral nerves and lymph nodes. Soft tissue calcification may occur either as amorphous masses or upon an ordered collagenous matrix as ectopic bone. This distinction is obvious histologically and can usually be made on a radiograph by the demonstration of trabeculation.

The prevalence of soft tissue calcification is unknown but it is certainly not rare. Indeed, calcification at certain sites, for example the costal cartilages (75% of all adults: Navani et al. 1970) or ligamentum nuchae, is so common in otherwise healthy individuals that it may be considered physiological. Calcification at other soft tissue sites is usually pathological and may be a feature of a number of diseases.

The diseases which may result in amorphous soft tissue calcification may be classified according to pathogenesis (Table 1.1). Customarily, three pathogenetic groups are distinguished: metastatic, dystrophic and idiopathic. Metastatic

Table 1.1. Soft tissue calcification: classification by pathogenesis.

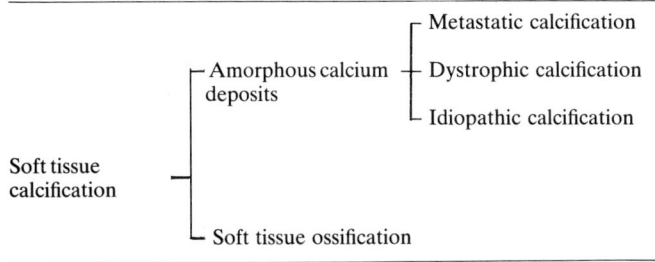

calcification may occur in any condition which produces a sustained elevation of the circulating levels of either calcium or phosphate so that the calcium phosphate product is elevated (Table 1.2). Calcification then occurs in previously normal tissues, characteristically the skin, subcutaneous tissue, periarticular tissues, blood vessels, corneae, conjunctivae and viscera. Such calcification is usually bilateral and fairly symmetrical.

Table 1.2. Causes of metastatic calcification.

Hypercalcemia
Hyperparathyroidism (primary or tertiary)
Sarcoidosis
Metastatic bone disease
Non-metastatic manifestation of malignant disease
Vitamin D intoxication
Milk–alkali syndrome
Paget's disease with immobilization

Hyperphosphatemia
Chronic renal failure
Hypoparathyroidism
Tumoral calcinosis (idiopathic hyperphosphatemia)

Table 1.3. Causes of dystrophic calcification.

Inherited
Ehlers–Danlos syndrome
Pseudoxanthoma elasticum
Alkaptonuria
Homocystinuria
Rothmund syndrome
Werner syndrome

Acquired
Blunt trauma
Thermal injury
Inflammation (of any cause)
Injection sites
Parasitic calcification
Dermatomyositis
Scleroderma (localized or systemic)
CRST syndrome
Lupus erythematosus (discoid or systemic)
Mixed connective tissue disease
Sarcoidosis
Atherosclerosis
Tumor calcification
Non-traumatic rhabdomyolysis

Dystrophic calcification occurs in areas of damaged soft tissue in the presence of normal levels of serum calcium and phosphate. The initial damage to the soft tissues may result from a number of diverse agents (Table 1.3). Calcification is localized to the site of injury and thus tends to be asymmetrical. There remains a group of diseases in which amorphous calcium deposits occur in apparently previously normal tissues in the presence of normal serum levels of calcium and phosphate (Table 1.4). This group has often been called idiopathic calcinosis, a term best avoided since it has been used indiscriminately in the older literature on ectopic calcification.

The presence of true bone in the soft tissues indicates a different group of diseases, as outlined in Table 1.5. If the lesion has a trabecular structure on a

Table 1.4. Idiopathic soft tissue calcification.

Calcific peritendinitis
Calcific bursitis
Chondrocalcinosis
Calcinosis circumscripta
?Calcinosis universalis
Monckeberg medial sclerosis
Phleboliths

Table 1.5. Causes of soft tissue ossification.

Post-traumatic ossification
Single major or repeated minor trauma; hematoma ossification; after hip replacement, burns, tetanus, surgical incisions

Tumor ossification
Parosteal osteosarcoma; soft tissue osteosarcoma; lipoma; skeletal muscle hemangioma; other connective tissue tumors; heterotopic bone-forming metastases; pseudomalignant myositis ossificans

Ossification in neurological conditions
Paraplegia; quadriplegia; hemiplegia; poliomyelitis; prolonged coma; neuropathic arthropathy

Fibrodysplasia ossificans progressiva

Other conditions
Ankylosing spondylitis; seronegative spondyloarthritides; diffuse idiopathic skeletal hyperostosis; ossification of the posterior spinal ligament; bridging of lumbar transverse processes; XYY syndrome; chronic venous insufficiency; osteoma cutis; hypoparathyroidism; stiff man syndrome; melorheostosis; localized progressive myositis ossificans; hereditary hypophosphatemia

radiograph (Figs. 1.1 and 1.2) then the differential diagnosis lies amongst these conditions. However, trabeculation will not be evident in the initial calcification of ectopic bone and may be poorly defined in an ossifying neoplasm. In these instances the initial differential diagnosis needs to include all causes of calcification for the affected area. Similarly, radio-opaque substances other than calcium salts may mimic amorphous tissue calcification and will need to be excluded in the absence of trabecular architecture.

In the diagnostic process, clues may be gathered at each stage of the patient's evaluation.

History

In the majority of diseases which may cause amorphous soft tissue calcification, symptoms and signs relate predominantly to the primary disease and the actual calcifications are asymptomatic. Occasionally skin or subcutaneous calcification may cause itching or may ulcerate through the skin and discharge chalky, white material. Infrequently amorphous calcification produces obvious soft tissue masses. This is most often seen after dermatomyositis or with tumoral calcinosis

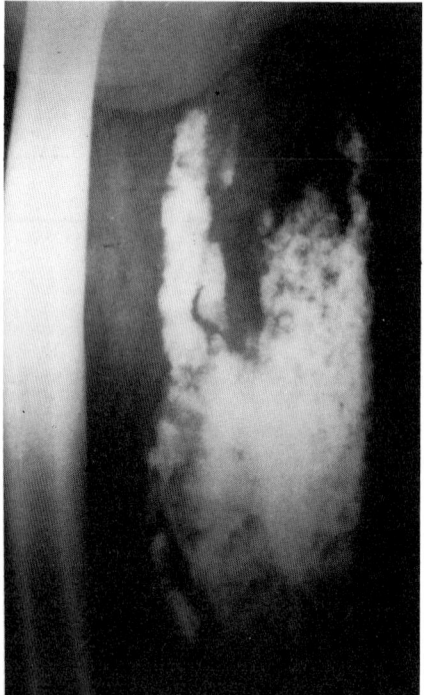 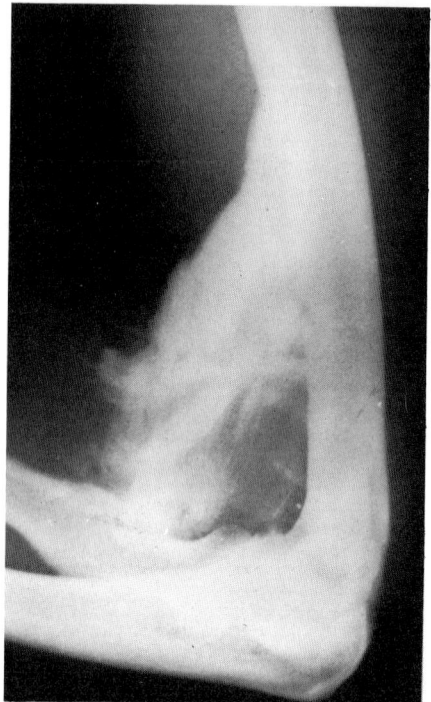

Fig.1.1. (*left*) Amorphous calcification in the soft tissues.
Fig.1.2. (*right*) Soft tissue ossification.

and is rare in other causes of metastatic calcification (Walker et al. 1977, Suzuki et al. 1979).

The symptoms of these primary disease processes which can cause amorphous soft tissue calcification (Tables 1.2–1.4) are covered in standard texts and need not be reviewed here, but a number of points deserve emphasis. The patient should be specifically asked about ingestion of milk and alkalis. A history of local injections, especially with calcium salts, epinephrine, quinine, opiates or bismuth (an old antisyphilitic: Fig. 1.3), should be sought as the patient may not realize its significance or may be reticent about volunteering information about the last two. Implantation calcification may occur at electroencephalogram electrode sites if paste containing calcium chloride is used (Wiley and Eaglestein 1979). Similar implantation has been reported in the skin abrasions of coal miners where the roof water contained a high concentration of calcium salts (Sneddon and Archibald 1958). This mechanism may help to explain obscure cases of skin calcification.

Calcification after dermatomyositis only occurs after several months or years. This delay may lead the clinician to overlook the significance of the original illness, especially when this was mild or non-specific. Many of the published cases of idiopathic calcinosis universalis undoubtedly represent calcification secondary to dermatomyositis or other collagen–vascular disorders, and there is some doubt about the existence of truly idiopathic calcinosis universalis (Wheeler et al. 1952, Hudson and Jones 1974).

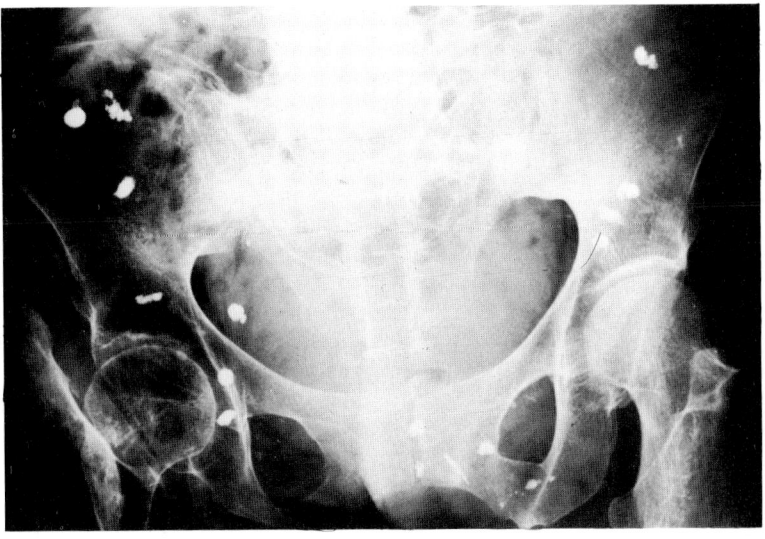

Fig.1.3. Multiple injections of bismuth in the treatment of syphilis.

Most clinicians are familiar with ossification after a major injury. Three points need to be stressed. First, this only follows a significant local injury, often sufficient to cause adjacent joint dislocation. Second, clinical and radiological evidence of ossification will be present within 2 months of the injury and ossification does not progress after 12 months. Finally the vast majority of lesions involve the muscles of the proximal limbs or the masseters. If the ossification is atypical in any of these respects, the diagnosis of post-traumatic ossification (syn. myositis ossificans traumatica) should be questioned. Multiple episodes of ossification after trauma should always raise the possibility of fibrodysplasia ossificans progressiva.

Tumors of soft tissue, either benign or malignant, present with an enlarging lump which may or may not be painful. Growth is usually progressive but is rarely so rapid as that seen in the development of an area of post-traumatic ossification. A vague or distant history of trauma is common in patients with ossifying tumors and in patients with pseudomalignant myositis ossificans, although its etiological significance is dubious (van der Heul and von Ronnen 1967, Ogilvie-Harris and Fornasier 1980).

Pseudomalignant myositis ossificans (syn. idiopathic myositis ossificans circumscripta) results in a solitary circumscribed area of soft tissue ossification which stops growing after 8 weeks and is usually found in the muscles of the thigh, mid-arm or hand. If the ossification is atypical in site or growth pattern then this diagnosis must be re-considered.

In contrast to amorphous calcification, soft tissue ossification usually produces local symptoms although the true nature of these may not be appreciated. Common symptoms include local pain and swelling with reduced mobility at adjacent joints. These symptoms may simulate an inflammatory process such as cellulitis, septic arthritis or superficial thrombophlebitis or, especially in paralysed patients, deep vein thrombosis may be suspected. Local pain is not invariable and will not be a feature in patients with complete cord transection. Some patients have no local symptoms except for insidious loss of joint motion and in others the ectopic bone is an unexpected finding on an incidental radiograph.

The patient's age is helpful in the differential diagnosis. Soft tissue calcification is rare in the first decade. Most cases in infancy are secondary to intravenous administration of calcium salts or subcutaneous fat necrosis and only occasionally due to congenital fibromatosis or idiopathic infantile arterial calcification (Ramamurthy et al. 1975, Shackleford et al. 1975, Propst-Proctor et al. 1982). In older children amorphous soft tissue calcification most commonly follows dermatomyositis or is due to tumoral calcinosis. Fibrodysplasia ossificans progressiva is the commonest cause of ectopic ossification in the first decade. In the second and third decades of life ectopic ossification is usually the result of trauma; pseudomalignant myositis ossificans is much less frequent. In the older age groups tumor ossification tends to predominate, whereas amorphous soft tissue calcification is usually the result of collagen–vascular or degenerative diseases.

The family history may provide important clues. Parental consanguinity or similarly affected siblings would suggest an autosomal recessive trait and in this context tumoral calcinosis, pseudoxanthoma elasticum, alkaptonuria, homocystinuria, and the Rothmund syndrome should be considered. Involvement of parent and child would suggest a dominant trait, either autosomal or X-linked, and pseudohypoparathyroidism, the Ehlers–Danlos syndrome and fibrodysplasia ossificans progressiva should be excluded. As individuals with the last-named disorder rarely reproduce, most patients represent fresh dominant mutations. The risk of such a dominant mutation increases with increasing paternal age and so age of the father at the birth of the child might be a clue to this disease.

Ethnic background may suggest the diagnosis. Tumoral calcinosis appears to be especially common in blacks (McClatchie and Bremner 1969) and ossification of the posterior longitudinal ligament of the spine attains a maximal prevalence amongst Japanese (Chin and Oon 1979). Parasitic infestation is endemic in certain areas of the world and parasitic calcification should be excluded in patients with a history of residence in one of these areas. For example, Reddy et al. (1968) noted calcified guinea worms in 4.6% of all radiographs taken at a hospital in Southern India. Fluorosis results in extensive ligamentous calcification and should be considered particularly in patients from the Punjab, Aden and South Africa.

Finally, the patient's occupation or recreational activities may provide the key to the diagnosis. Horse-riding may result in ossification of the thigh adductors; drill bones occur in the pectorals and deltoids of infantrymen; the thigh muscles ossified in old-fashioned cobblers; and participants in contact sports are liable to post-traumatic ossification (Smith 1960). Calcification of the ischiogluteal bursae is an occupational hazard for seamstresses (Withersty and Chillag 1979).

Physical Examination

Conjunctival deposits of calcium appear as greyish granules at the corneoscleral junction and suggest metastatic calcification. Skin and subcutaneous calcification is often apparent upon palpation and may be evident before radiographs are abnormal. Similarly, pinnal calcification and ossification is easily overlooked unless the external ear is routinely palpated (McKusick and Goodman 1962).

Dystrophic calcification may be suggested by the presence of skin changes of scleroderma, systemic lupus erythematosus, pseudoxanthoma elasticum or the Ehlers–Danlos syndrome.

Local swelling, tenderness, warmth and adjacent joint limitation may be features of the early stages of ectopic ossification. Later, a hard mass is apparent which may be fixed deeply but not to the overlying skin (Fig. 1.4). Loss of joint

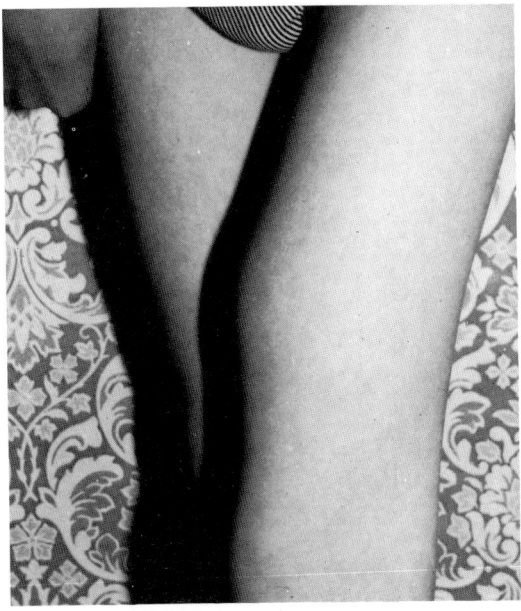

Fig.1.4. Soft tissue swelling due to ectopic ossification.

movement may range from none to complete ankylosis. The discovery of a hard calcified mass in the soft tissues always raises the question of neoplasia (Fig. 1.5; Clair and Majumudar 1980): this and other differential diagnoses are outlined in Table 1.6.

Ossifying tumors usually present with a single lump which is progressive in size and may be painful. Synovial sarcoma is usually periarticular (Wright et al. 1982). Soft tissue osteosarcoma most commonly arises in the thigh muscles and parosteal osteosarcoma typically arises in the popliteal fossa. Compression of local nerves or vessels is not a feature of pseudomalignant myositis ossificans or fibrodysplasia ossificans progressiva and would favor a neoplasm.

Tumoral calcinosis causes lobulated masses about the hip, shoulder and elbow; these masses may become enormous. In both this and the calcification secondary to dermatomyositis multiple calcified lumps are usual. Ossifying tumors and pseudomalignant myositis ossificans are generally solitary. Multiple ossifying lumps are usually due to fibrodysplasia ossificans progressiva; occasionally ossifying metastatic disease is responsible.

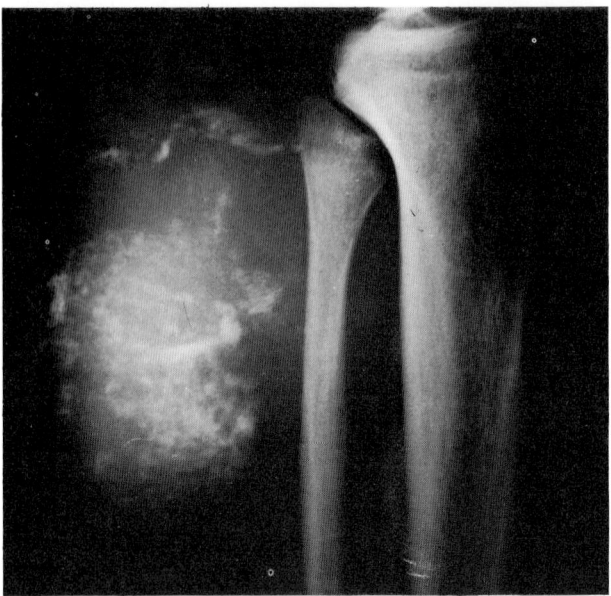

Fig.1.5. Amorphous calcification in a fibrosarcoma.

Table 1.6. Differential diagnosis of a calcified soft tissue mass.

Mass with amorphous calcification

Benign
Early stages of an ossifying lesion; dermatomyositis; tumoral calcinosis; parasitic calcification; metastatic calcification; injection granuloma; lipoma; hemangioma; chondroma

Malignant
Synovial sarcoma; chondrosarcoma; fibrosarcoma; liposarcoma; hemangiosarcoma; hemangiopericytoma; sweat gland carcinoma; malignant breast tumor

Mass with ossification

Benign
Post-traumatic ossification (myositis ossificans); ossification secondary to hip replacement, surgical scars, neurological conditions, burns or tetanus; fibrodysplasia ossificans progressiva; lipoma; skeletal muscle hemangioma; benign mesenchymoma; pseudomalignant myositis ossificans; localized progressive myositis ossificans; bony exostosis; massive callus; dysplasia epiphysealis hemimelica

Malignant
Parosteal osteosarcoma; soft tissue osteosarcoma; malignant mesenchymoma; osteosarcoma of bone with soft tissue invasion; heterotopic bone-forming metastases; rhabdomyosarcoma; sacrococcygeal teratoma; malignant breast tumor

---

Fibrodysplasia ossificans progressiva should be suspected if a child has any of the following features: neck stiffness, short thumbs or malformed big toes. The abnormal big toes are usually noted at birth and differ radiologically from isolated congenital hallux valgus.

Shortened metacarpals may be a feature of pseudohypoparathyroidism.

Laboratory Tests

Normal levels of serum calcium and phosphate will exclude metastatic calcification (Table 1.2). Serum alkaline phosphatase may be elevated during the early stages of ectopic ossification of any cause. This is not invariable and although an elevated alkaline phosphatase level would support the diagnosis of ectopic ossification, a normal level would not exclude it. The elevation of alkaline phosphatase when due to ectopic ossification is caused by increase of the bone isoenzyme.

Levels of creatine phosphokinase and other muscle enzymes will be abnormal during the active phase of dermatomyositis but are usually normal by the stage of soft tissue calcification.

An elevated erythrocyte sedimentation rate is not a feature of ectopic ossification and might suggest a collagen–vascular disorder, in which case a variety of autoantibodies might be sought.

Eosinophilia may be marked in patients with parasitic infestation.

Radiology

Plain radiographs, especially xeroradiographs, help to identify and localize soft tissue calcification (Tables 1.7–1.10). In many cases the radiographic appearance is sufficiently characteristic for a definitive diagnosis to be made. This will apply to atheromatous calcification, phleboliths, Monckeberg medial sclerosis, ankylosing spondylitis, diffuse idiopathic skeletal hyperostosis, calcific peritendinitis, post-injection densities, chondrocalcinosis, and most cases of parasitic calcification (Fig. 1.6).

Table 1.7. Skin and subcutaneous fat calcification.

Common causes
Burns; chronic venous insufficiency; metastatic calcification; dermatomyositis; scleroderma; CRST syndrome; fat necrosis; injection sites; acne vulgaris; surgical incisions

Rare causes
Ossifying skin tumors; systemic lupus erythematosus; rheumatoid arthritis; pseudoxanthoma elasticum; Ehlers–Danlos syndrome; lipoma; Rothmund syndrome; epidermolysis bullosa; primary osteoma cutis; sarcoidosis; Werner syndrome; Weber–Christian disease

Table 1.8. Skeletal muscle and tendon calcification.

Common causes
Calcific peritendinitis; post-traumatic ossification; ossification in neurological conditions; dermatomyositis; parasitic calcification; injection sites

Rare causes
Pseudomalignant myositis ossificans; fibrodysplasia ossificans progressiva; post-pyogenic myositis; post carbon monoxide poisoning; scleroderma; skeletal muscle hemangioma; hemophilia; Volkmann's contracture; soft tissue osteosarcoma; heterotopic bone-forming metastases

Table 1.9. Periarticular calcification.

Common causes

Post-traumatic ossification; ossification after joint replacement; chondrocalcinosis; metastatic calcification; scleroderma; CRST syndrome; dermatomyositis; burns; calcific bursitis; ankylosing spondylitis; diffuse idiopathic skeletal hyperostosis; seronegative spondyloarthritides; ossification in neurological conditions

Rare causes

Synovial sarcoma; synovial chondromatosis; fibrodysplasia ossificans progressiva; alkaptonuria; melorheostosis; gout; tuberculosis; hypervitaminosis A; fluorosis; post-pyogenic arthritis; hereditary hypophosphatemia

---

Table 1.10. Calcification at other soft tissue sites.

Intra-articular calcification

Bone fragments (trauma, osteochondromatosis); chondrocalcinosis; metastatic calcification; post-traumatic calcification; post-pyogenic arthritis; idiopathic intervertebral disc calcification; synovioma; calcific synovitis; intracapsular chondroma

Vascular calcification

Atherosclerosis; diabetes mellitus; metastatic calcification; phleboliths; homocystinuria; Monckeberg medial sclerosis

Peripheral nerve calcification

Leprosy; neurofibromatosis

Calcification of lymph nodes

Tuberculosis; histoplasmosis; coccidiodomycosis; *Filaria bancrofti*; post-BCG inoculation; metastases; malignant lymphoma after radiotherapy; silicosis; sarcoidosis

Calcification of the pinna

Frostbite; Addison's disease; acromegaly; diabetes mellitus; metastatic calcification; syphilitic perichondritis; alkaptonuria; trauma; familial cold hypersensitivity; diastrophic dysplasia; systemic chondromalacia; hypopituitarism; hyperthyroidism; pseudohypoparathyroidism; sarcoidosis; old age

---

Calcification after dermatomyositis occurs in muscle fascial planes, skin and subcutaneous tissue, especially of the proximal limbs, pelvic girdle, trunk and neck (Steiner et al. 1974, Sewell et al. 1978, Fig. 1.7). It is the leading cause of extensive soft tissue calcification. Occasionally calcification after systemic lupus erythematosus may be as extensive (Weinberger et al. 1979). Idiopathic calcinosis universalis, if it exists, would also produce such a picture. Extensive calcification which is restricted to the legs is most commonly due to subcutaneous ossification secondary to chronic venous insufficiency. Strauss and Harari (1977) described a similar radiographic picture in an 83-year-old Russian who had repeatedly injected his legs with kerosene in an attempt to avoid conscription to the Czarist army.

In scleroderma, powdery punctate and large discrete densities are present in the fingers and over pressure points (Schlenker et al. 1973). Systemic lupus erythematosus may mimic this pattern (Bundin and Feldman 1975). These collagen–vascular disorders account for many cases of localized skin calcification: some, however, remain unexplained and these are lumped under the descriptive title of idiopathic calcinosis circumscripta (Greenfield 1980).

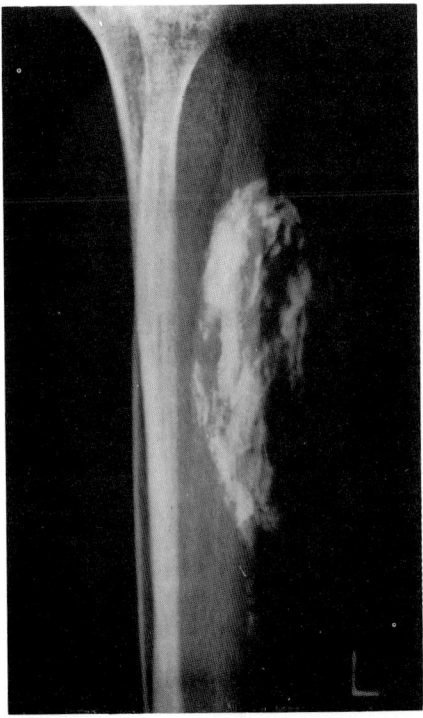 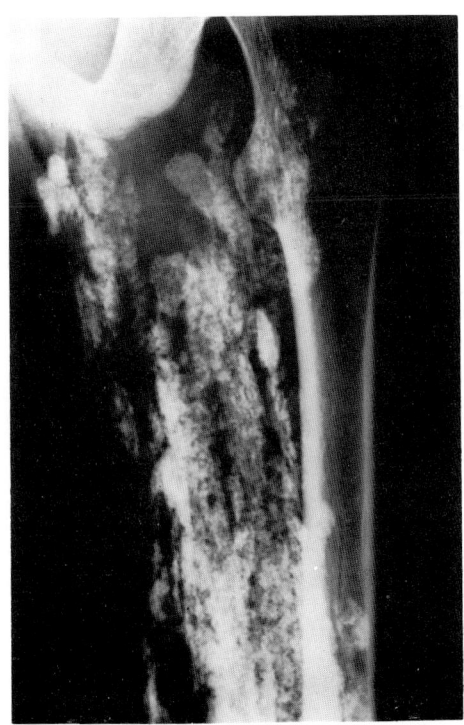

Fig.1.6. (*left*) Dystrophic calcification of a tuberculous ulcer.
Fig.1.7. (*right*) Amorphous soft tissue calcification following dermatomyositis.

Metastatic calcification typically produces pipe-stem arterial calcification and deposits about joints, in skin and in viscera, especially the kidney. The periarticular deposits in tumoral calcinosis may become enormous and as the contents are semi-fluid a fluid level may be seen (Hug and Gunçaga 1974, Fig. 1.8). Rarely other causes of metastatic calcification may produce similar large periarticular masses (Walker et al. 1977, Suzuki et al. 1979, Feldman et al. 1981).

Regardless of its actual cause an area of ectopic ossification has a distinctive radiological course. Initially, there is soft tissue swelling which then develops diffuse calcification. Subsequently, mature trabeculated bone is seen (Figs. 1.9 and 1.10).

Pseudomalignant myositis ossificans is characterized by a lucent zone between the lesion and the underlying bone, an intact underlying cortex, diaphyseal location, dense peripheral calcification and loss of volume on serial films (Goldman 1976).

Soft tissue osteosarcoma is commonest in the thigh and contains variable streaky radio-opacities. If the adjacent bone is invaded this will result in a saucerized defect which helps to distinguish this lesion from a primary osteosarcoma of bone with secondary soft tissue invasion (Greenfield 1980).

Parosteal osteosarcoma arises from the metaphysis of a bone, typically the distal femur, tends to encircle the bone with a 1 to 3 mm gap, and has characteristic radiolucent areas which correspond to areas of fibrous tissue and cartilage.

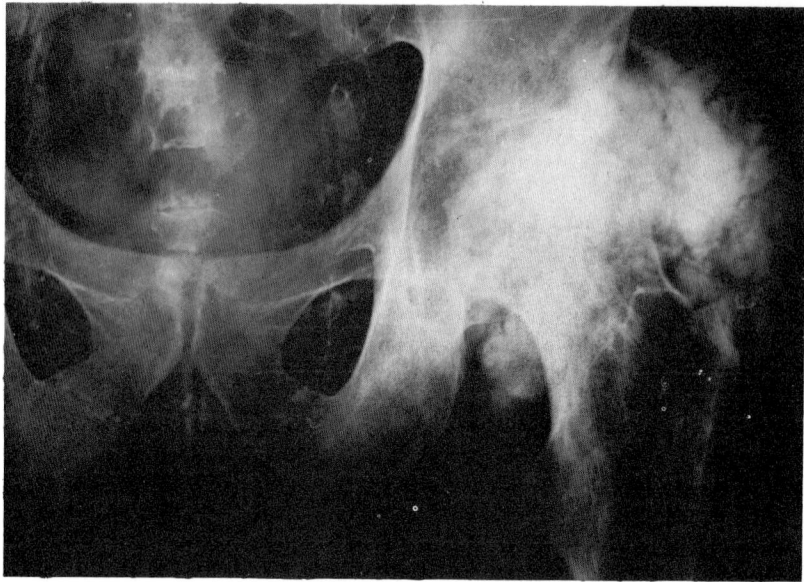

Fig.1.8. Periarticular and vascular calcification in tumoral calcinosis.

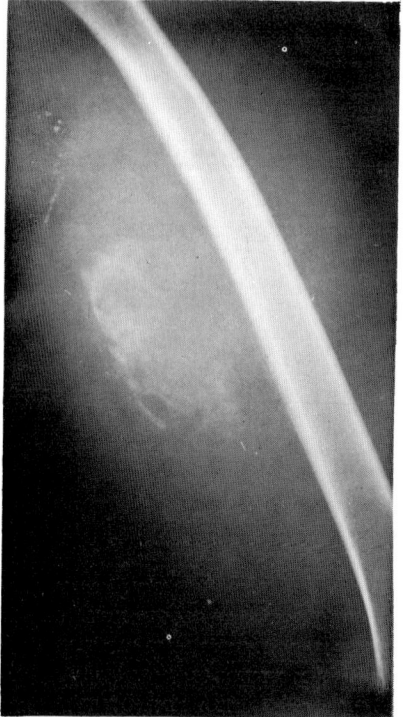 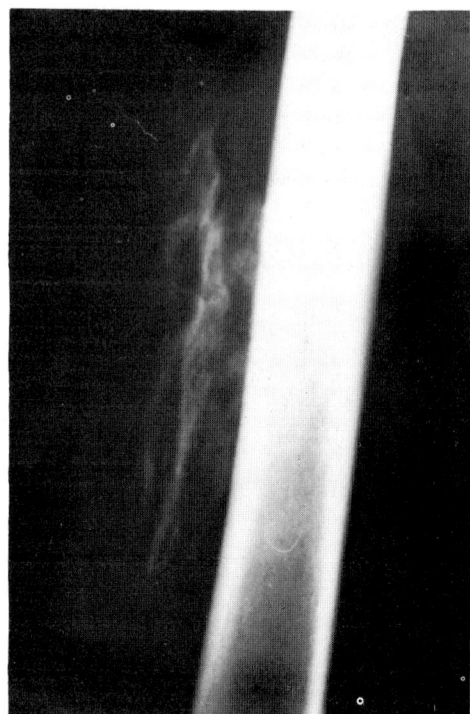

Fig.1.9. (*left*) Early ectopic ossification.
Fig.1.10. (*right*) Mature ectopic bone.

Fibrodysplasia ossificans progressiva is almost invariably the diagnosis in a patient with widespread ectopic ossification. Certain skeletal malformations are common findings in this condition. These include: short first metacarpals, hypoplastic middle phalanges of the fifth fingers, malformed phalanges of the big toes, abnormal first metatarsals, short, broad femoral necks, metaphyseal spurs and abnormal cervical vertebrae. As the disease progresses cervical fusion is frequent and these changes in the neck may be mistaken for the Klippel–Feil syndrome or juvenile rheumatoid arthritis (Connor and Smith 1982).

Plain radiographs also permit the diagnosis of conditions which may simulate a soft tissue ossifying lump, such as a primary osteosarcoma of bone which has invaded the soft tissues, hyperplastic callus in osteogenesis imperfecta, a bony exostosis and dysplasia epiphysialis hemimelica.

The radiologist will thus be able to provide a definite diagnosis for many cases of soft tissue calcification.

Angiography

In the active stage of pseudomalignant myositis ossificans there are numerous fine vessels which result in a diffuse stain; later the lesion is usually avascular. In contrast, malignant tumors typically show pathological vessels, arteriovenous shunts, venous lakes, amputated vessels, invasion of large arteries and veins, and large abnormal draining veins (Hutcheson et al. 1972, Yaghmai 1977). In addition to aiding the differential diagnosis, angiography may be helpful in planning surgical resection of a soft tissue tumor.

Bone Scan

Scanning with 99m technetium is strongly positive in all types of soft tissue calcification and ossification (Richards 1974, Akmal et al. 1978, Leicht et al. 1979). This reflects the similarity of the mineral component of bone and of amorphous calcification. Newly formed crystal tends to dissolve and re-crystallize spontaneously. At this stage radionuclides can exchange for ions in newly formed mineral and the uptake depends upon blood supply and mineral turnover of the area. This technique is thus of no use in the differential diagnosis of these conditions although it may be useful for assessing the extent of involvement, and serial scans will aid the assessment of activity in an area of ectopic bone. Further, with ectopic ossification a bone scan will be positive before mineral is apparent on plain radiographs and thus is very helpful for early diagnosis.

Computerized Tomography

The technique of computerized tomography allows a precise localization of the site of ectopic calcification and often reveals calcifications which are not visible on plain radiographs (Vas et al. 1981). Its value in aiding the differential diagnosis of calcified soft tissue masses has yet to be fully exploited.

Ultrasound

There have been few published reports on the use of ultrasound in the evaluation of calcified soft tissue masses. Kramer et al. (1979) used ultrasound on a girl with pseudomalignant myositis ossificans and noted a soft tissue mass with a bright reflector indicating calcification.

Biopsy

In the majority of patients with soft tissue calcification, biopsy will not be required in order to make the diagnosis.

In post-traumatic ossification with typical clinical and radiological features, biopsy is unnecessary and may delay recovery (Tredget et al. 1977). Similarly biopsy is unnecessary for diagnosing ossification after tetanus, burns, neurological lesions or hip replacement.

In the author's experience, a biopsy in the early stages of fibrodysplasia ossificans progressiva is frequently misinterpreted as fibrosarcoma, lipofibrosarcoma or congenital fibromatosis. Furthermore the biopsy often produces an exacerbation of ossification and thus should be avoided since a firm diagnosis of this condition can be made on the basis of the clinical and radiological findings.

Likewise, a diagnosis of pseudomalignant myositis ossificans can usually be made without a biopsy. Ogilvie-Harris and Fornasier (1980) also make the point that, if biopsy is undertaken, a needle biopsy is undesirable as, if only the central zone is sampled, a misdiagnosis of malignancy is likely.

Biopsy is mandatory where a calcifying or ossifying soft tissue neoplasm is suspected or cannot be otherwise excluded. Histopathological classification of these tumors is comprehensively covered in several specialized texts (Dahlin 1978, Schajowicz 1981) and is briefly discussed in Chap. 3.

Summary

The diagnosis in the vast majority of patients with soft tissue calcification will be possible on the basis of history, physical examination, routine biochemical tests and plain radiographs. Bone scanning has a role in early diagnosis and assessment of activity of ectopic ossification. Patients with a calcified or ossified soft tissue neoplasm will require biopsy for definitive diagnosis. In the future computerized tomography will probably play an increasingly important part in the assessment of calcified soft tissue masses.

References

Akmal M, Goldstein DA, Telfer N, Wilkinson E, Massry SG (1978) Resolution of muscle calcification in rhabdomyolysis and acute renal failure. Ann Intern Med 89: 928–930

Bundin JA, Feldman F (1975) Soft tissue calcifications in systemic lupus erythematosus. AJR 124: 358–364

Chin WS, Oon CL (1979) Ossification of the posterior longitudinal ligament of the spine. Br J Radiol 56: 865–869

Clair JTSt, Majumudar B (1980) Tumoral calcinosis masquerading as metastatic carcinoma. Gynecol Oncol 10: 69–74

Connor JM, Evans DAP (1982) Fibrodysplasia ossificans progressiva. The clinical features and natural history of 34 patients. J Bone Joint Surg [Br] 64: 76–83

Connor JM, Smith R (1982) The cervical spine in fibrodysplasia ossificans progressiva. Br J Radiol 55: 492–496

Dahlin DC (1978) Bone tumors, 3rd edn. Charles C Thomas, Springfield, Illinois

Feldman ES, Dalinka MK, Schumacher HR (1981) Diffuse soft tissue calcification in tumoral calcinosis. Skeletal Radiol 7: 33–35

Goldman AB (1976) Myositis ossificans circumscripta: A benign lesion with a malignant differential diagnosis. AJR 126: 32–40

Greenfield GB (1980) Radiology of bone diseases, 3rd edn. JB Lippincott Co, Philadelphia Toronto

Hudson PM, Jones PE (1974) Extensive calcinosis with minimal scleroderma: Treatment of ectopic calcification with aluminium hydroxide. Proc R Soc Med 67: 1166–1168

Hug I, Gunçaga J (1974) Tumoral calcinosis with sedimentation sign. Br J Radiol 47: 734–736

Hutcheson J, Klatte EC, Kremp R (1972) The angiographic appearance of myositis ossificans circumscripta. A case report. Radiology 102: 57–58

Kramer FL, Kurtz AB, Rubin C, Goldberg BB (1979) Ultrasound appearance of myositis ossificans. Skeletal Radiol 4: 19–20

Leicht E, Berberich R, Lauffenburger T, Haas HG (1979) Tumoral calcinosis: Accumulation of bone-seeking tracers in the calcium deposits. Eur J Nucl Med 4: 419–421

McClatchie S, Bremner AD (1969) Tumoral calcinosis—an unrecognised disease. Br Med J i: 153–155

McKusick VA, Goodman RM (1962) Pinnal calcification: Observations in systemic diseases not associated with disordered calcium metabolism. JAMA 179: 230–232

Navani S, Shah JR, Levy PS (1970) Determination of sex by costal cartilage calcification. AJR 108: 771–774

Ogilvie-Harris DJ, Fornasier VL (1980) Pseudomalignant myositis ossificans: Heterotopic bone formation without history of trauma. J Bone Joint Surg [Am] 62: 1274–1283

Propst-Proctor SL, Jones RB, Nagel DA (1982) Iatrogenic soft-tissue calcification in an extremity. J Bone Joint Surg [Am) 64: 449–450

Ramamurthy RS, Harris V, Pildes RS (1975) Subcutaneous calcium deposition in the neonate associated with intravenous administration of calcium gluconate. Pediatrics 55: 802–806

Reddy CRRM, Sivaprasad MD, Parvathi G, Chari PS (1968) Calcified guinea worm: Clinical, radiological and pathological study. Ann Trop Med Parasitol 62: 399–406

Richards AG (1974) Metastatic calcification detected through scanning with 99mTc polyphosphonate. J Nucl Med 15: 1057–1060

Schajowicz F (1981) Tumors and tumorlike lesions of bones and joints. Springer, New York Heidelberg Berlin

Schlenker JD, Clark DD, Weckesser EC (1973) Calcinosis circumscripta of the hand in scleroderma. J Bone Joint Surg [Am] 55: 1051–1056

Sewell JR, Liyanage B, Ansell BM (1978) Calcinosis in juvenile dermatomyositis. Skeletal Radiol 3: 137–143

Shackleford GD, Barton LL, McAlister WH (1975) Calcified subcutaneous fat necrosis in infancy. J Can Assoc Radiol 26: 203–207

Smith ET (1960) Myositis ossificans of the humerus (Blocker's disease). Texas J Med 56: 678–680

Sneddon IB, Archibald RML (1958) Traumatic calcinosis of the skin. Br J Dermatol 70: 211–214

Steiner RM, Glassman L, Schwartz MW, Vanace P (1974) The radiological findings in dermatomyositis of childhood. Radiology 111: 385–393

Strauss S, Harari Z (1977) Extensive bilateral lower leg calcification in an elderly man. JAMA 238: 431–432

Suzuki K, Takahashi S, Ito K, Tanaka Y, Sezai Y (1979) Tumoral calcinosis in a patient undergoing hemodialysis. Acta Orthop Scand 50: 27–31
Tredget T, Godberson CV, Bose B (1977) Myositis ossificans due to hockey injury. Can Med Assoc J 116: 65–66
van der Heul RO, von Ronnen JR (1967) Juxtacortical osteosarcoma. Diagnosis, differential diagnosis, treatment and an analysis of eighty cases. J Bone Joint Surg [Am] 49: 415–439
Vas W, Cockshott WP, Martin RF, Pai NK, Walker I (1981) Myositis ossificans in hemophilia. Skeletal Radiol 7: 27–31
Walker GS, Davison AM, Peacock M, McLachlan MSF (1977) Tumoral calcinosis: A manifestation of extreme metastatic calcification occurring with 1,alpha-hydroxycholecalciferol therapy. Postgrad Med J 53: 570–573
Weinberger A, Kaplan JG, Myers AR (1979) Extensive soft tissue calcification (calcinosis universalis) in systemic lupus erythematosus. Ann Rheum Dis 38: 384–386
Wheeler CE, Curtis AC, Cawley EP, Grekin RH, Zheutlin B (1952) Soft tissue calcification with special reference to its occurrence in the 'collagen diseases'. Ann Intern Med 36: 1050–1075
Wiley HE 3rd, Eaglestein WE (1979) Calcinosis cutis in children following electroencephalography. JAMA 242: 455–456
Withersty DJ, Chillag SA (1979) Seamstress's bottom. Am Fam Physician 19: 85
Wright PH, Sim FH, Soule EH, Taylor WF (1982) Synovial sarcoma. J Bone Joint Surg [Am] 64: 112–122
Yaghmai I (1977) Myositis ossificans: Diagnostic value of arteriography. AJR 128: 811–816

2 Ossification After Major Trauma

Skeletal muscle ossification after a single major injury is one of the commonest causes of soft tissue ossification. Although the clinical features are characteristic, there was little attempt to distinguish this from other causes of soft tissue ossification until the beginning of this century (Binnie 1903, Finney 1910, Painter 1921).

The name traumatic myositis ossificans has been widely used in the older literature. However, this term is inappropriate as muscles are not invariably involved and the lesions are not inflammatory in nature (Gilmer and Anderson 1959). Other synonyms include myositis ossificans traumatica, traumatic ossifying myositis, myo-osteosis, extra-osseous localized non-neoplastic bone and cartilage, and heterotopic bone formation.

Prevalence

Otto (1816) is believed to have described the first patient with post-traumatic ossification and by 1910 more than 150 case reports had appeared in the literature (Finney 1910). Several large series followed and by 1914 more than 500 patients had been described (Oliver 1914).

In the past, the kicks of horses were the commonest source of trauma but in recent years these have been surpassed by sports injuries and road traffic accidents.

The site of injury is an important factor. Ectopic ossification is a classic complication of injuries to the elbow. Thompson and Garcia (1967) noted ossification in 35 (8%) of 447 patients with traumatic dislocation of the elbow. Similarly it may occur in up to 15% of patients with traumatic dislocation of the hip, especially if open reduction is required (Paus 1951, Hunter 1969). The thigh muscles are also a common site for post-traumatic ossification, but the exact prevalence at this site is unknown.

Clinical Features

Ossification after trauma is predominantly a disease of adolescent and young adult males, with only occasional reports in other age groups and females (Ellis and Frank 1966, Wilkes 1976). The limb muscles are usually affected and brachialis, quadriceps or the thigh adductors are by far the commonest sites of involvement

(Gruca 1925). The distal parts of the limbs are uncommonly involved, with only four reports of post-traumatic ossification in the hand despite the frequency of trauma to this area (Mallory 1933, Duncan 1974, Johnson and Lawrence 1975, Altner and Singh 1981). The muscles of mastication may ossify after trauma and 15 cases have been reported up to 1980 (Mulherin and Schow 1980). Thirteen of these involved the masseters, with one each in the medial pterygoid and suprahyoid muscles. Post-traumatic ossification of other muscles appears to be rare.

The frequency of ossification seems to be related to the severity of the initial injury. Thus, Thompson and Garcia (1967) noted ectopic bone in 11 (4%) of 311 patients with elbow dislocation alone compared with 24 (18%) of 136 patients with fracture-dislocation of the elbow (Fig. 2.1). Curiously, only a proportion of individuals with equally severe injuries at a certain site will develop ectopic bone. This observation led several authors to suggest an individual predisposition to ossification after trauma (Painter 1921, Campbell 1934, Thorndike 1940). Furthermore, a patient with a previous episode of post-traumatic ossification seems to be at increased risk for ossification at other sites if subjected to future episodes of trauma (Tredget et al. 1977).

Ossification of the soft tissues should be suspected if pain, swelling and local tenderness persist after an injury. Local warmth may be marked and suggest an inflammatory process although systemic features such as fever are not seen. Both active and passive movements will be reduced and as the pain gradually subsides, a circumscribed indurated, and later hard, mass is palpable.

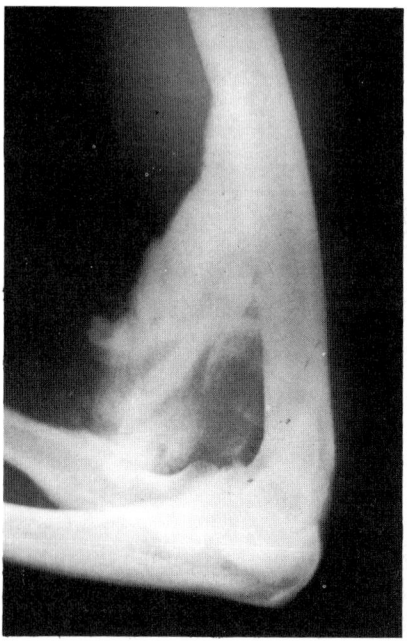

Fig. 2.1. Ectopic ossification following elbow dislocation.

During the convalescent phase of a quadriceps lesion, the patient may have a characteristic limp and be referred to by athletics coaches as a 'Charley horse'. Charley was apparently an old white horse with a marked limp which belonged to the Sioux City baseball team in the 1890s (Lloyd et al. 1936).

Compression of local nerves or vessels is rarely a feature of post-traumatic ossification. Jones and Ward (1980) described bilateral ossification in the biceps femoris muscles which was ascribed to trauma sustained during weight-lifting. This led to a left sciatic palsy which resolved with excision of the ossified mass. Similarly, Kleiman et al. (1971) noted compression of the sciatic nerve by ectopic ossification after a fracture-dislocation of the hip. The ipsilateral facial palsy in the patient with masseteric ossification reported by Shawkat (1967) was probably a direct result of the original injury. Likewise, the sciatic palsy in the patient described by Thakkar and Porter (1981) was a direct result of fracture-dislocation of the hip. The subsequent ectopic bone surrounded the sciatic nerve as a tube but did not result in neurological compression.

Total white cell count, erythrocyte sedimentation rate, and serum calcium, phosphate and alkaline phosphatase levels are within normal limits.

Radiology

The radiographic evolution of post-traumatic ossification parallels the histological pattern (Norman and Dorfman 1970). Shortly after the injury, soft tissue swelling is evident. By 3–4 weeks, flocculated densities are present in the mass which have been likened to cotton-candy. A periosteal reaction of the underlying bone may be seen but a radiolucent zone separates the lesion from the underlying periosteal reaction and cortex. A lacy pattern of new bone is present at 6–8 weeks and the mass is sharply circumscribed peripherally by a cortex (Fig. 2.2). The mass shrinks

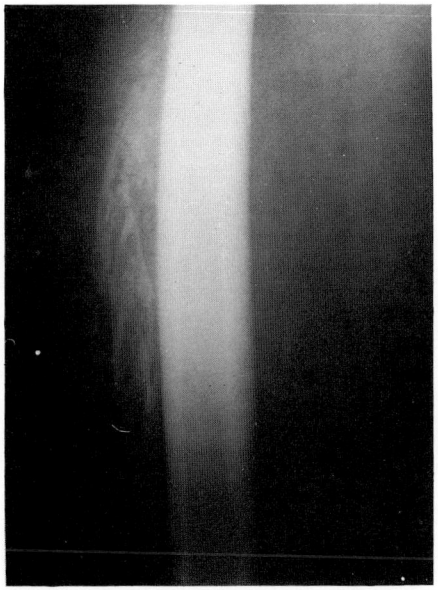

Fig.2.2. Ectopic bone 8 weeks after blunt thigh injury.

radiologically mature bone with well-marked trabeculation by 5–6 months
2.3). At this stage the lesion may become attached to the underlying normal
(Greenfield 1980).

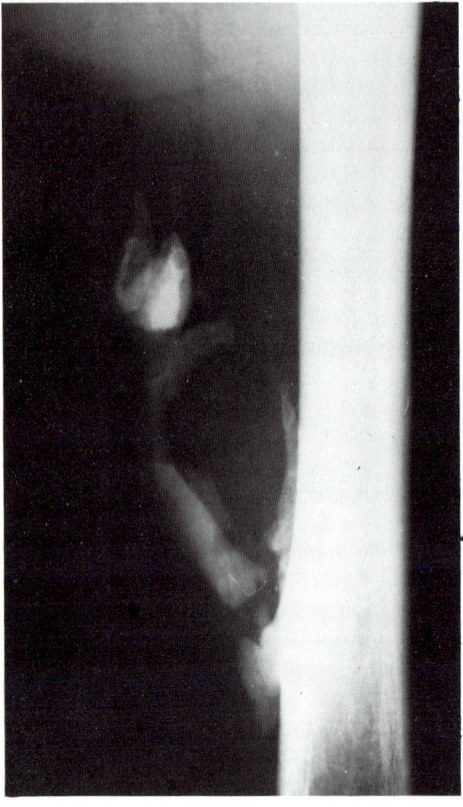

Fig.2.3. Ectopic bone 1 year after blunt thigh injury.

Pathology

As early surgery almost invariably leads to recurrence, most histopathological studies have concerned the later stages of this disease (Geschickter and Maseritz 1938, Gilmer and Anderson 1959).

A striking proliferation of undifferentiated mesenchymal cells occurs within 3–4 days of the injury. There is marked local edema at this stage but neither hematoma nor inflammation are features. In the absence of the clinical history, a biopsy of the lesion during this early proliferative phase may be difficult, if not impossible, to distinguish from a sarcoma. Bone is found within the lesion by 3–4 weeks and although foci of cartilage (Fig. 2.4) are often seen in the intervening period it is believed that most bone forms by intramembranous ossification (Bona et al. 1967, Pinter et al. 1980).

It is uncertain from the published literature whether the zonal phenomenon of centrifugal maturation which is so typical of pseudomalignant myositis ossificans (see p. 46) is also seen in post-traumatic ossification (Gilmer and Anderson

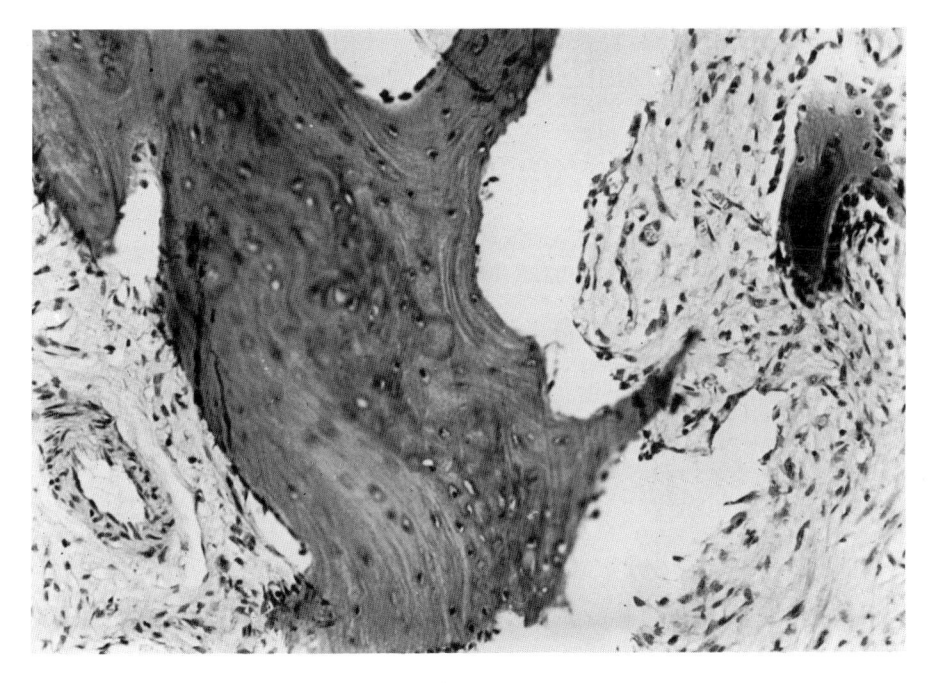

Fig.2.4. Histopathology of ectopic bone secondary to trauma (H and E, ×150).

1959). However, in experimental post-traumatic ossification in rabbits a zonal phenomenon is marked, there being inner undifferentiated proliferating mesenchymal cells, a middle zone of osteoid and outer maturing bone (Michelsson et al. 1980).

Ossification after major trauma is usually clinically obvious and ideally biopsy should be avoided as it is liable to stimulate further ossification and delay recovery (Tredget et al. 1977).

Pathogenesis

Older theories of pathogenesis included: ossification of a hematoma, periosteal damage leading to release of periosteal osteoblasts, or activation of periosteal osteoblasts which were already in the muscle. Ossification in a muscle hematoma can occur but is very rare and has a distinctive radiological and pathological appearance (see p. 24). Periosteal damage is not seen at operation nor is it a prerequisite in experimental animals.

Recent studies (see p. 112), however, have clearly shown the existence of cells in the connective tissues of experimental animals which, under appropriate circumstances, can differentiate into osteoblasts. These cells are known as inducible osteogenic precursor cells (IOPC), and although found in several types of connective tissue are especially frequent in the connective tissue of skeletal muscles. They are believed to be the source of the ectopic osteoblasts in post-traumatic ossification and other forms of ectopic ossification. The mechanism by which trauma can activate the IOPC and the reason why some individuals seem prone to such activation with trauma are unknown. Furthermore, the characteristic involvement of some muscles and the sparing of others, remains a mystery.

Natural History

When an area of post-traumatic ossification is not removed, it gradually matures and usually becomes orientated in the direction of adjacent muscle fibers. Often it becomes covered with cartilage and later fusion of the new bone with the underlying cortex can occur.

Most lesions persist indefinitely but some will completely disappear. Thorndike (1940) reported a prolonged follow-up on 25 patients with post-traumatic ossification. In 9 (36%) the lesions resorbed spontaneously. This was especially likely with small lesions and was commoner in the arm than the leg, except for ectopic bone in the region of the elbow. Spontaneous resorption may be more frequent in younger patients (Thompson and Garcia 1967, Dickerson 1971). Even if the ectopic bone persists, the overall prognosis is good for the recovery of full painless movement (Ellis and Frank 1966).

A recurrent question with regard to post-traumatic ossification has been the possibility of malignant transformation. This issue has been confused by the problems of interpretation of early histological features. Some patients with 'benign' myositis ossificans have had needless surgery or radiotherapy for presumed sarcoma. Conversely, in other patients a lesion initially interpreted as myositis ossificans behaved as though it were malignant from the outset (Shanoff et al. 1967, Järvi et al. 1968). In many patients with proven osteosarcoma of bone or soft tissue osteosarcoma there is often a vague or distant history of trauma which is of dubious etiological importance (van der Heul and von Ronnen 1967). As mentioned earlier, ossification after a single major trauma occurs, by definition, directly after a significant injury. In such cases of post-traumatic ossification there have been a few reports where an area of ectopic bone was stable for some years but subsequently increased in size and on biopsy was malignant (Geshickter and Maseritz 1938, Pack and Braund 1942—case 1, Kagan and Steckel 1978). Thus ectopic bone is not immune from malignant transformation but considering the frequency of post-traumatic ossification the risk of this complication appears to be no higher than for the normal skeleton.

Management

Management can be considered in two parts: the treatment of established ectopic ossification and prophylaxis.

In the early stages of post-traumatic ossification the limb should be rested and elevated. Local heat, massage and range of motion exercises should be avoided at this stage. As pain and swelling subside, active range of motion exercises can be started and eventually, progressive resistance exercises can be introduced to restore muscle strength (Jackson and Feagin 1975).

Early excision of ectopic bone is contra-indicated as it almost invariably leads to locally extensive recurrent ossification (Thorndike 1940). Excision of persistent ectopic bone is only indicated for persistent pain, muscle weakness or serious joint limitation (Lipscomb et al. 1976). Surgery should be deferred for 6–12 months until the lesion is mature as evidenced by a stable radiological appearance and decreasing isotope uptake on serial bone scans. Despite these precautions recurrence is frequent after excision of post-traumatic ectopic bone from the region of the hip or the elbow (Epps 1978). Thompson and Garcia (1967) obtained a good result in only 1 of 8 patients in whom they excised bone from the region of the elbow. Auto-transplantation of fat has been successfully used to prevent re-ossification following excision of ectopic bone after hip replacement (Riska and Michelsson 1979) and deserves evaluation in the prevention of recurrence after excision of post-traumatic ectopic bone.

Radiotherapy, ultrasound, short-wave diathermy, hyaluronidase, corticosteroids and proteolytic enzymes are ineffective in the treatment of post-traumatic ossification. Radiotherapy may actually be harmful since it carries a small, but definite, increased risk of osteosarcoma of the irradiated bone and soft tissues (Chap. 3).

At the present time, there is no proven means of preventing soft tissue ossification after single major injury. This condition is certainly common enough to permit the organization of double-blind trials of potential prophylactic agents or regimes.

Ossification After Repeated Minor Trauma

Soft tissue ossification can also follow episodes of repeated minor trauma. Invariably, connective tissue of muscles or tendons is involved and the individual episodes of trauma are in themselves mild and often forgotten. By virtue of their occupational or recreational activities certain individuals incur such repeated episodes of trauma and the sites of involvement are quite characteristic (Table 2.1).

Fout and McLeod (1977) reported ossification in the left deltoids of two US sailors after repeated punches to the area. This appears to be the price of success and reflects the tradition adopted from the British navy of 'tacking on the crow'. When a sailor attains promotion his new stripe is tacked on by the fist blows of his peers. In both of these cases the ectopic bone was excised without recurrence.

Table 2.1. Ectopic ossification after repeated minor trauma.

Occupation/recreation	Site of ossification	Comment
Horse-riding	Thigh adductors	Rider's bone Prussian's disease
Cavalry	Outer side of thigh	Secondary to repeated scabbard contact
Infantry/rifle-shooting	Pectoral and deltoid muscles	Drill bones
Fencing	Brachialis	
Ballet	Gastrocnemius	
Old-fashioned cobbling	Thigh muscles	At site of contact with shoe last

Again not all individuals develop ectopic bone despite similar repetitive trauma. Coley (1913) commented that drill bones were present in 18 (3%) of 600 conscripts who had been exposed to repeated musket recoil.

Ossification may also occur at sites of repeated narcotic injection, either intramuscular or failed intravenous injections, and this led Deutsch (1971) to coin the term 'drug abusers elbow'. Such ossification in the antecubital fossa has been successfully excised (Chung 1973). Similarly, in the past ossification was occasionally noted at sites of repeated intramuscular injection of quinine used in the treatment of malaria (Severi 1933). Ossification at injection sites needs to be distinguished from amorphous calcification and from the injection of other radio-opaque substances such as bismuth (Chap. 1).

Hematoma Ossification

Zadek (1969) reported a patient whose hematoma had undergone ossification. Radiologically, the lesion had a well-defined ovoid appearance and was remote from bone (Fig. 2.5). At operation, a thin shell of ossification surrounded a central area of old hemorrhage: features which are quite distinct from those seen in post-traumatic ossification (see p. 17). Zadek could find no similar cases in a review of the world literature for the preceding 25 years. Thus ossification within a hematoma, as opposed to amorphous calcification, would appear to be a rare event. Certainly in clinical practice, the vast majority of hematomas resolve spontaneously and completely.

If hematomas were a common site for ossification then soft tissue ossification should be a frequent occurrence in patients with hemorrhagic diatheses. After

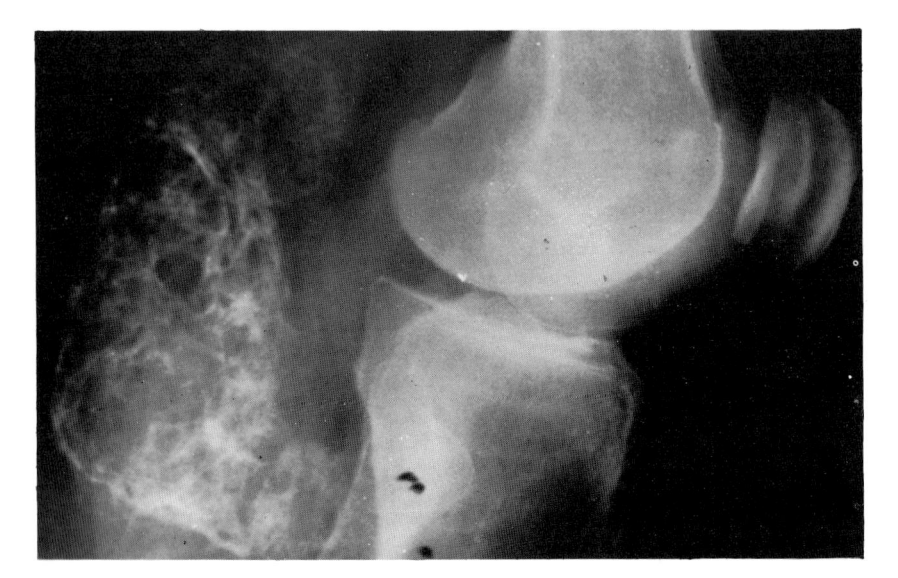

Fig.2.5. Ossification of a hematoma.

joint hemorrhage, intramuscular hemorrhage is the commonest site for spontaneous hemorrhage in classical hemophilia (factor VIII deficiency) (Goodfellow et al. 1967). However, ectopic ossification in hemophiliacs is uncommon and to date only 17 instances have been reported (Petersen 1947, Sampinato 1970, Hutcheson 1973, Heim et al. 1979, Vas et al. 1981). These ossifications are typically in the peripelvic area, especially in iliopsoas and the thigh adductors. No specific treatment has been required.

Peripelvic soft tissue ossification has also been described in a female who was treated with anticoagulants for thrombophlebitis (Sampinato 1970). Another patient, described by Jokl and Federico (1977), who had partial factor XI deficiency and multiple areas of ossification, had an additional risk factor in that he was a college football halfback.

Post-traumatic Ossification of Ligaments and Tendons

The collagenous tissue of many large tendons in adults undergoes a transition to fibrocartilage. Ossification may follow either single major or repetitive minor trauma at certain sites as described below. Similar ossifications are a common finding in certain animal species, especially fowl (Abdalla 1979).

Achilles Tendon Ossification

Achilles tendon ossification was first reported in 1908 by Horing and by 1970, 30 cases had been described (Lotke 1970). The age range has been wide and the youngest patient to date was 9 years old at diagnosis. Males predominated, in the ratio of 2:1.

Most patients are asymptomatic and if pain occurs a fracture through the ossified mass should be suspected. Clinically a hard tender mass is present in the Achilles tendon, usually at its junction with the muscle belly or at its insertion into the calcaneus, and the true nature of the lesion is revealed by X-ray (Figs. 2.6 and 2.7).

More than one half of patients had a history of trauma or surgery to the tendon (Ghormley 1938). Usually the surgery involved was subcutaneous tenotomy and surprisingly no cases have been described following formal Achilles tendon lengthening (Brotherton and Ball 1979).

If the condition is asymptomatic, no treatment is necessary. If painful, the mass should be excised to relieve symptoms and to prevent tendon rupture (Fisher and Woods 1970, Lotke 1970).

Patellar Tendon Ossification

Ossification of the patellar tendon may follow major or repeated minor injuries to the tendon. Since Osgood–Schlatter's disease is also related to stress transmitted to the tibial tubercle by this tendon it is common for the two to coexist (Cole 1937). A familial factor may be involved since 3 of the 24 patients reported by Cole (1937) had similarly affected family members. Local symptoms are usually absent but if

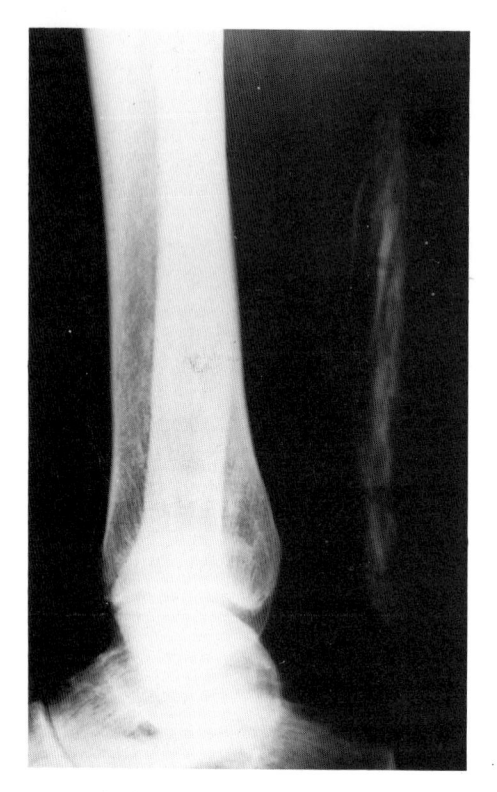

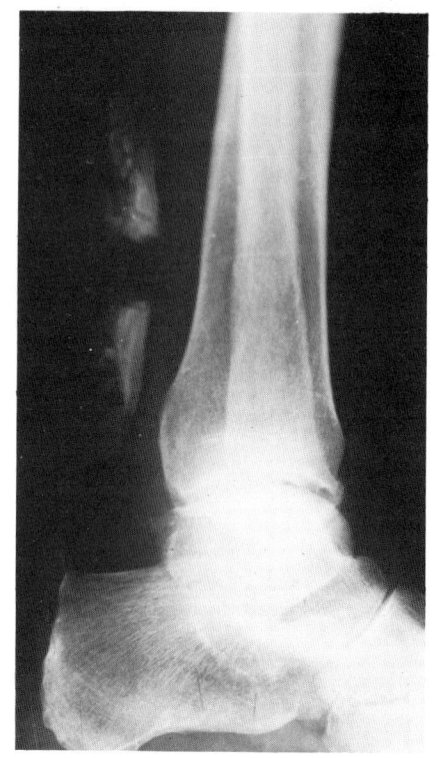

Fig.2.6. (*left*) Ossification of Achilles tendon.
Fig.2.7. (*right*) Fracture of ectopic bone in Achilles tendon.

present local injection with hydrocortisone may be beneficial (Holstein et al. 1964). Occasionally, excision of the ossified area from the tendon will be necessary.

Re-emphasizing the similarity of ectopic to normal bone, Hadjipavlou et al. (1981) described the changes of Paget's disease in an area of ectopic bone in the left patellar tendon and in the adjacent skeleton.

Pellegrini–Stieda Disease

Post-traumatic calcification of the medial collateral knee ligament was first described by Kohler in 1903 and was subsequently delineated by Pellegrini in 1905 and Stieda in 1908. By 1938 Pellegrini was able to find 767 cases in the world literature. Thus this is a common disorder although the exact prevalence is not known.

The initiating knee injury may be mild or severe. Frequently, the patient is asymptomatic, but if radiographed about 3 weeks after the injury, calcification in the medial collateral ligament is apparent. Occasionally, persistent discomfort is noted but usually there are no clinical abnormalities. The calcific deposit increases in density and size over the next few weeks and then stabilizes. Ossification, which often follows, may remain confined to the ligament or may gain an attachment to the femoral condyle. Infrequently, similar changes may occur in the lateral collateral ligament.

Early manipulation should be avoided and other treatment is usually unnecessary (Houston et al. 1968).

Ossification of the Anterior Longitudinal Ligament of the Cervical Spine

In contrast to ossification of the posterior longitudinal ligament (see p. 91), ossification of the anterior longitudinal ligament of the cervical spine is usually secondary to neck trauma (Bailey and Kato 1972). Schneider et al. (1962) described this as an occupational hazard in the divers of Acapulco who make daily dives from over 35 m. Usually patients are asymptomatic but compression of the esophagus leading to dysphagia may occur (Khalifa et al. 1981). Diagnosis is established by the typical location of the ossification and treatment is usually unnecessary.

Ossification After Hip Replacement

Prevalence

All major series have noted ectopic ossification after hip replacement. The prevalence varied widely from 8% to 90% (Table 2.2). Some of this wide range reflects differing criteria for diagnosis and the fact that minor degrees of ossification are often overlooked. Kromann-Andersen et al. (1980) prospectively assessed 309 patients after hip replacement and noted 49% affected at 3 months,

Table 2.2. Ectopic ossification after hip replacement.

Series	No. of operations	Any ossification (%)	Clinically serious ossification (%)
Amstutz (1970)	50	8	2
Hamblen and Harris (1971)	422	20	3
Charnley (1972)	379	ns	5
Brooker et al. (1973)	100	21	2
Lazansky (1973)	501	8	0.5
Nollen and Slooff (1973)	200	53	7
Matos et al. (1975)	221	41	13
DeLee et al. (1976)	2173	15	ns
Riegler and Harris (1976)	102	50	2
Salvati et al. (1976)	100	39	3
Rosendahl et al. (1977)	117	90	15
Beckenbaugh and Ilstrup (1978)	333	ns	5
Slätis et al. (1978)	145	37	ns
Mollan (1979)	131	18	ns
Kromann-Andersen et al. (1980)	309	71	ns

ns, not stated.

61% at 2 years and 71% at 5 years. Thus the variable duration of follow-up must also be considered when comparing different series.

Risk Factors

In most series there has been an excess of affected males, often with a sex ratio of 2–3 males to 1 female (DeLee et al. 1976, Kromann-Andersen et al. 1980), but in occasional series females predominated (Riegler and Harris 1976). The age range of the patients who develop this complication does not appear to differ from that of those who do not, but there does appear to be an individual predisposition. In the large series of DeLee et al. (1976), 22 of 295 patients with a history of previous hip surgery (excluding replacement) had developed soft tissue ossification. All 22 developed ectopic bone with subsequent joint replacement. DeLee et al. (1976) also found that if one side was affected after hip replacement there was a 92% chance of ossification after replacement of the opposite hip, as compared with an expected incidence of 14.6%. Likewise, the majority of patients with concurrent bilateral hip replacements who develop soft tissue ossification do so bilaterally although usually asymmetrically (Nollen and Slooff 1973, Kromann-Andersen et al. 1980).

The very high prevalence of 90% reported by Rosendahl et al. (1977) reflects the large number of patients who developed ossification in the region of the greater trochanter and these authors suspected that this was due to the need to strip the periosteum from this region during McFarland's approach. Otherwise the type of operation or choice of prosthesis does not appear to influence ectopic ossification (Ritter and Vaughan 1977). No difference has been noted between elective and acute surgery.

The patient's primary disease which resulted in the need for hip replacement may be a factor but the available evidence is conflicting (Table 2.3). Ectopic ossification may be more frequent if the patient has either ankylosing spondylitis or prominent marginal osteophytes (Lazansky 1973, DeLee et al. 1976, Ritter and Vaughan 1977). Osteophytes are a prominent feature of diffuse idiopathic skeletal hyperostosis (DISH) and DISH may also be an important risk factor (Resnick et

Table 2.3. Ectopic ossification after hip replacement according to primary disease.

Series	No. of operations	Primary disease[a]	Any ossification (%)	Clinically serious ossification (%)
Taylor et al. (1976)	150	OA	37	4
	150	RA	21	0
	70	AS	49	9
DeLee et al. (1976)	ns	OA	16	ns
	ns	RA	11	ns
	ns	AS	6	ns
	ns	CDH	12	ns
Bisla et al. (1976)	23	AS	62	ns
Stauffer and Sim (1976)	35	Paget's	ns	23

ns, not stated.
[a] OA, osteoarthrosis; RA, rheumatoid arthritis; AS, ankylosing spondylitis; CDH, congenital dislocation of the hip.

al. 1976, Blasingame et al. 1981). Both DISH and ankylosing spondylitis have been associated with HLA B27 in various studies (see p. 87); thus studies of histocompatibility antigens in patients who develop this complication after hip replacement may help to define the patient at risk. To date there have been few studies in this area. Mattingly and Mowat (1980) found no HLA association in 16 patients with ectopic ossification after hip replacement for osteoarthrosis.

Mollan (1979), in a prospective study, suggested that there was a group of patients with pre-operative elevations of serum alkaline phosphatase who were prone to soft tissue ossification. In Paget's disease, however, the level of pre-operative alkaline phosphatase bears no relation to the incidence of ectopic ossification (Stauffer and Sim 1976).

Experience with replacement of joints other than the hip is more limited. Soft tissue ossification appears to be a less frequent complication of knee replacement than of hip replacement (Booth and King 1979).

The high-risk patient would appear to be a male with a primary disease characterized by ectopic ossification who had ossification after replacement of the opposite hip.

Clinical Features

Typically the patient has normal progress to about the 6th week after surgery and then develops increased hip pain, slight swelling and progressive limitation of active and passive movements. Clinically serious loss of function occurs in 0.5%–15% of patients after hip replacement (Table 2.2). Those with functional impairment have extensive ectopic bone or ankylosis (Brooker et al. 1973). The remainder have few or no local symptoms, in which case the area of ossification is an incidental radiological finding.

The results of routine laboratory tests, including serum calcium and phosphate levels, muscle enzyme levels and erythrocyte sedimentation rate, are within normal limits. The serum alkaline phosphatase is inconstantly elevated around the 3rd week after operation and is generally normal by the time ectopic bone is present on radiographs (Nollen and Slooff 1973, Mollan 1979).

Radiology

Radiological evidence of ossification may be apparent as early as 3 weeks after the operation as irregular mottled opacities (Rosendahl et al. 1977). Most cases are, however, detected at 6–12 weeks post-operation. The extent of such ossification can be conveniently assessed using the classification proposed by Brooker et al. (1973) (Table 2.4). DeLee et al. (1976) noted that 28% of lesions were radiologically mature at 6 months and 72% at 12 months.

Pathology

Most commonly the ectopic bone forms in the hip abductors (Riegler and Harris 1976). The sequence of pathological changes seems to resemble that described for post-traumatic soft tissue ossification but again there is a lack of serial studies since most lesions are mature when excised.

2.4. Classification of ossification after hip replacement.

Grade I	Islands of bone within soft tissues about hip
Grade II	Bone spurs from pelvis or proximal end of femur, leaving at least 1 cm between opposing bone surfaces
Grade III	As grade II but gap less than 1 cm
Grade IV	Apparent bony ankylosis of the hip

After Brooker et al. (1973).

Pathogenesis

There are many similarities between the ossification after hip replacement and that seen after blunt trauma to the tissues, and similar pathogenetic theories have been proposed to explain both. Ossification in local hematomata appears unlikely, as this is not seen pathologically and does not account for the lack of this complication after other, equally hemorrhagic, operations. Rosendahl et al. (1977) favor metaplasia of local connective tissue cells from the perimysium and endomysium. Cells with the potential to become osteoblasts, the inducible osteogenic precursor cells, are now known to be a normal component of the connective tissue of muscles and tendons in experimental animals (see p. 112). It is suspected, but not yet proven, that the situation in man is similar and that these cells are responsible for ectopic bone production. However, the mechanism by which surgery activates these cells remains a mystery. Certainly local infection, as suggested by Amstutz (1970), is not the activating agent (Ritter and Vaughan 1977). In addition, the reason why certain individuals seem to be unduly susceptible to this complication is not understood.

Natural History

Functional impairment occurs in only a small fraction of patients (Brooker et al. 1973). Untreated, the ectopic ossification usually persists, but DeLee et al. (1976) found no cases where soft tissue ossification either appeared or increased in amount after the first post-operative year.

Management

Treatments may be divided into two groups: those concerned with established soft tissue ossification and prophylactic measures.

Excision offers the only hope of cure for those with established soft tissue ossification and obviously will only be required in those few patients who have significant functional impairment. There is a high risk of recurrence if the bone is excised before maturity. Thus a delay of at least 1 year is advised, the x-ray appearance should be stable, scrum alkaline phosphatase normal and there should be a decreasing uptake of isotope on serial bone scans. Despite these precautions many patients still have recurrence (Epps 1978). The report of Riska and Michelsson (1979) that bone did not recur during prolonged follow-up on 6 patients after excision with auto-transplantation of fat to the excision site thus merits further evaluation. Medications, such as corticosteroids or diphosphonates, are ineffective against established ectopic ossifications.

The diphosphonates, and especially disodium etidronate (EHDP), have been evaluated for the prophylaxis of soft tissue ossification. In vitro and in experimental animals, this group of compounds inhibits mineralization of bone matrix (Francis et al. 1969). Unfortunately, this therapy does not appear to prevent formation of the ectopic bone matrix; the incidence and extent of radiological ossification is decreased whilst on therapy, but after EHDP is stopped, ectopic mineral is promptly deposited. Thus EHDP does not prevent, but merely delays the deposition of calcium in the ectopic bone matrix (Nollen and Slooff 1973, Bijvoet et al. 1974). Seven patients of DeLee et al. (1976) developed soft tissue ossification whilst on systemic corticosteroids for their primary joint disease.

Coventry and Scanlon (1981) recently reported on the use of radiotherapy in the management of ectopic ossification after hip replacement. They concluded that this form of treatment was of no value for established ectopic ossification but seemed to reduce the incidence and severity of ectopic bone if used prophylactically. These conclusions were, however, based on an uncontrolled trial, and in experimental animals and other forms of human soft tissue ossification radiotherapy has not been shown to have any prophylactic value.

At the present time there is thus no established means of prophylaxis of this complication of hip replacement.

Ossification After Burns

Prevalence

Ossification as a complication of burns was first described by Johnson in 1957. Boyd et al. (1959) surveyed 1000 children with burns severe enough to require hospitalization and found 6 with ossification. It may be more common in adults, as Evans (1966) found that 29 (2%) of 1460 hospitalized burns patients were affected. Munster et al. (1972) in a prospective study of patients with burned arms found ossification in the region of the elbow in 11% and Schiele et al. (1972) in a similar prospective study found an incidence of 23% (16) in 70 patients. In recent years, however, parallelling the progress in early mobilization of patients with burns, the incidence of this complication appears to have fallen (Evans 1978).

Clinical Features

Affected patients usually have a full thickness skin loss of 22% or more (Evans 1966). Soft tissue ossification is usually recognized at 3–7 months after the burn, when one or more joints is found to be stiff. Lesions are usually periarticular but the anatomical distribution of the burn does not dictate the localization of the ectopic bone. In adults the elbow is most commonly involved, followed by the shoulder and rarely the hip, whereas in children the hip and elbow are affected with equal frequency (Evans 1966). Of the 29 patients detected by Evans (1966), 24 had limitation of joint movements and 11 had changes at more than one joint. Bilateral elbow involvement was particularly frequent. Restriction of joint movement may precede radiographic changes (Hoffer et al. 1978).

Serum calcium, phosphate and alkaline phosphatase levels are within normal limits.

Radiology

Initial radiological changes consist of an amorphous cloudy mass with subsequent maturation to lamellar bone. Schiele et al. (1972) in a prospective radiographic study noted these changes most commonly about the elbow, but similar findings were also present in the proximal and distal parts of the interosseous membrane and adjacent to the ulnar styloid.

Pathology

The histology of early lesions is not known but the mature lesions consist of histologically normal bone, complete with osteoblasts, osteocytes, osteoclasts, Haversian systems and marrow. Posterior osseous bridging from the olecranon to the medial epicondylar ridge of the humerus is the typical lesion in adults. In children, however, anterior bridging of the elbow is more frequent. The other sites of involvement include brachialis, biceps, the medial border of triceps, subscapularis, gluteus medius, gluteus minimus and iliopsoas. The articular surfaces of extensively involved joints will eventually be lost and intra-articular ankylosis will ensue.

Pathogenesis

The occurrence of ossification is related to the extent of the initial burn. In addition to the tissue damage burns patients are subjected to a period of functional immobility. This period of confinement is also a factor and ossification was only seen by Evans (1966) in those patients who had been confined to bed for more than 2 months. This may account for the reduced incidence of this complication in recent years, which has coincided with the encouragement of early mobilization.

An individual predisposition is also suspected, since not all patients with burns of similar severity and similar periods of immobilization will develop this complication. This predisposition may be inherited, for Evans (1978) noted the occurrence of soft tissue ossification with much the same distribution in twin brothers, neither of whom was seriously burned.

Natural History

The areas of ossification may increase in size as long as there are open granulating areas or areas of proliferating scar tissue. If bridging of a joint occurs then the ectopic bone will persist indefinitely. If not, it will start to diminish in size once the skin lesions have healed and nitrogen equilibrium has been restored (Evans 1966). Ectopic bone may even resolve spontaneously, especially in children (Munster et al. 1972).

Management

In children, resection is rarely necessary as spontaneous recovery of motion is usual (Hoffer et al. 1978). In adults resorption is slow and operation may be required. Of the 29 adult patients studied by Evans (1966), 17 required surgery: all had functional improvement and none had any recurrence of ossification. Although excision is effective when bridging is limited to one plane, the prognosis for restoration of joint function is poor for bridging in more than one plane. In patients who, despite physiotherapy, have significant limitation of movement, excision may be performed as soon as the skin has healed (Evans 1978).

The encouragement of early mobilization would seem to be important in the prophylaxis of this complication.

Ossification After Tetanus

Prevalence

Ossification after tetanus was first reported by Gunn and Young in 1959. To date there have been less than 30 reported cases and this appears to be a rare complication of tetanus, even in countries where the disease is endemic (Odiase 1975).

Clinical Features

Most cases have been discovered about 4–8 weeks after the onset of the flexor spasms. During convalescence the patient notes limitation of one or more joints and a soft tissue mass may be palpable. The elbows are most commonly involved, followed by the shoulders, hips and knees (Mitra et al. 1976, Jajić and Rulnjević 1979). The results of routine hematological and biochemical tests are within normal limits.

Radiology

Radiologic changes are present at 4–7 weeks after the onset of tetanic convulsions (Femi-Pearse and Olowu 1971). The lesion gradually becomes more and more dense and finally may differentiate into cortex and medulla (Mitra et al. 1976).

Pathology

Nothing is known of the histopathology in the early stages. In the late stages where ectopic bone has been excised, mature lamellar bone has been found.

Pathogenesis

Most authors attribute these changes to trauma to the muscles from the tetanic spasms (Femi-Pearse and Olowu 1971). Odiase (1975), though, has pointed out that flexor muscles are not affected even though their contractions dominate the clinical picture.

Renier et al. (1966) described para-articular ossification, typical of that seen in neurological lesions (Chap. 5), in two patients who had been treated for tetanus by curarization and artificial ventilation. In these two patients the changes were believed to be secondary to prolonged immobilization rather than muscle trauma. Both factors, trauma and immobilization, may of course be involved, but again the mechanism by which they activate the inducible osteogenic precursor cells to become osteoblasts is unknown (see p. 108).

Natural History

If untreated, the ectopic bone appears to persist, but reported cases are few and follow-up is inadequate to give definite data on this point.

Management

The ectopic bone has been successfully excised in several patients, with restoration of function and without recurrence.

References

Abdalla O (1979) Ossification and mineralization in the tendons of the chicken (*Gallus domesticus*). J Anat 129: 351–359
Altner PC, Singh SK (1981) An unusual case of ectopic ossification in a finger. J Hand Surg 6: 142–145
Amstutz HC (1970) Complications of total hip replacement. Clin Orthop 72: 123–137
Bailey HL, Kato F (1972) Paravertebral ossification of the cervical spine. South Med J 65: 189–192
Beckenbaugh RD, Ilstrup DM (1978) Total hip arthroplasty. J Bone Joint Surg [Am] 60: 306–313
Bijvoet OLM, Nollen AJG, Sloof TJJH, Feith R (1974) Effect of a diphosphonate on para-articular ossification after total hip replacement. Acta Orthop Scand 45: 926–934
Binnie JF (1903) On myositis ossificans traumatica. Ann Surg 38: 423–440
Bisla RS, Ranawat CS, Inglis AE (1976) Total hip replacement in patients with ankylosing spondylitis with involvement of the hip. J Bone Joint Surg [Am] 58: 233–238
Blasingame JP, Resnick D, Coutts RD, Danzig LA (1981) Extensive spinal osteophytosis as a risk factor for heterotopic bone formation after total hip arthroplasty. Clin Orthop 161: 191–197
Bona C, Stanescu V, Dumitrescu MS, Ionescu V (1967) Histochemical and cytoenzymological studies in myositis ossificans. Acta Histochem 27: 207–224
Booth CM, King JB (1979) Myositis ossificans following total knee replacement. A report of two cases. Arch Orthop Trauma Surg 93: 285–286
Boyd BM Jr, Roberts WM, Miller GR (1959) Periarticular ossification following burns. South Med J 52: 1048–1051
Brooker AF, Bowerman JW, Robinson RA, Riley LH Jr (1973) Ectopic ossification following total hip replacement. Incidence and a method of classification. J Bone Joint Surg [Am] 55: 1629–1632
Brotherton BJ, Ball J (1979) Fracture of an ossified Achilles tendon. Injury 10: 245–247
Campbell ER (1934) Traumatic myositis ossificans. South Med J 27: 763–769
Charnley J (1972) The long-term results of low-friction arthroplasty of the hip performed as a primary

References

intervention. J Bone Joint Surg [Br] 54: 61–76
Chung BS (1973) Drug-induced myositis ossificans circumscripta. JAMA 226: 469
Cole JP (1937) A study of Osgood–Schlatter disease. Surg Gynecol Obstet 65: 55–67
Coley WB (1913) Myositis ossificans traumatica. Ann Surg 57: 305–337
Coventry MB, Scanlon PW (1981) The use of radiation to discourage ectopic bone. A nine-year study in surgery about the hip. J Bone Joint Surg [Am] 63: 201–208
DeLee JG, Ferrari A, Charnley J (1976) Ectopic bone following low friction arthroplasty of the hip. Clin Orthop 121: 53–59
Deutsch I (1971) Myositis ossificans: Complication of drug abuse. JAMA 216: 1035
Dickerson RC (1971) Myositis ossificans in early childhood. Report of an unusual case. Clin Orthop 79: 42–43
Duncan AM (1974) Angiographic abnormalities in combined myositis ossificans and digital ischemia of the hand. Report of a case. Acta Radiol 15: 152–156
Ellis M, Frank HG (1966) Myositis ossificans traumatica: with special reference to the quadriceps femoris muscle. J Trauma 6: 724–738
Epps CH Jr (1978) Complications in orthopedic surgery. JB Lippincott Co, Philadelphia Toronto
Evans EB (1966) Orthopaedic measures in the treatment of severe burns. J Bone Joint Surg [Am] 48: 643–669
Evans EB (1978) Musculoskeletal changes complicating burns. In: Epps CH Jr (ed) Complications in orthopedic surgery. JB Lippincott Co, Philadelphia Toronto
Femi-Pearse D, Olowu AO (1971) Myositis ossificans—a complication of tetanus. Clin Radiol 22: 89–92
Finney JMT (1910) Myositis ossificans traumatica. South Med J 3: 36–45
Fisher TR, Woods CG (1970) Partial rupture of the tendo calcaneus with heterotopic ossification. Report of a case. J Bone Joint Surg [Br] 52: 334–336
Fout LR, McLeod TL (1977) Heterotopic ossification in the brachium secondary to unusual trauma. Milit Med 142: 622–623
Francis MD, Russell RGG, Fleisch H (1969) Diphosphonates inhibit formation of calcium phosphate crystals in vitro and pathological calcification in vivo. Science 165: 1264–1266
Geschickter CF, Maseritz IH (1938) Myositis ossificans. J Bone Joint Surg 20: 661–674
Ghormley JW (1938) Ossification of the tendo achillis. J Bone Joint Surg 20: 153–160
Gilmer WS Jr, Anderson LD (1959) Reactions of soft somatic tissue which may progress to bone formation: Circumscribed (traumatic) myositis ossificans. South Med J 52: 1432–1448
Goodfellow J, Fearn CBd'A, Matthews JM (1967) Iliacus hematoma. A common complication of haemophilia. J Bone Joint Surg [Br] 49: 748–756
Greenfield GB (1980) Radiology of bone diseases, 3rd edn. JB Lippincott Co, Philadelphia Toronto
Gruca A (1925) Myositis ossificans circumscripta. A clinical and experimental study. Ann Surg 82: 883–919
Gunn RD, Young WB (1959) Myositis ossificans as a complication of tetanus. J Bone Joint Surg [Br] 41: 535–540
Hadjipavlou A, Lander P, Boudreau R, Srolovitz H, Palayew M (1981) Pagetoid changes in a heterotopic center of ossification. A case report. J Bone Joint Surg [Am] 63: 1339–1341
Hamblen DL, Harris WH (1971) Myositis ossificans as a complication of hip arthroplasty. J Bone Joint Surg [Br] 53: 764
Heim MD, Strauss S, Horoszowski H (1979) Peripelvic new bone formation following saddle injuries in hemophiliac patients: Report of two cases. J Trauma 19: 846–847
Hoffer MM, Brody G, Ferlic F (1978) Excision of heterotopic ossification about elbows in patients with thermal injury. J Trauma 18: 667–670
Holstein A, Lewis GB, Schulze R (1964) Heterotopic ossification of patellar tendon. Bull Hosp Joint Dis 25: 191–200
Höring F (1908) Über Tendinitis ossificans traumatica. Münch Med Wochnschr 55: 674–675
Houston AN, Roy WA, Faust RA, Edwin DM, Espenan PA (1968) Pellegrini–Stieda syndrome: Report of 44 cases followed from original injury. South Med J 61: 113–117
Hunter GA (1969) Posterior dislocation and fracture-dislocation of the hip. A review of fifty-seven patients. J Bone Joint Surg [Br] 51: 38–44
Hutcheson J (1973) Peripelvic new bone formation in hemophilia. Report of three cases. Radiology 109: 529–530
Jackson DW, Feagin JA (1975) Quadriceps contusion in young athletes: Relation of severity of injury to treatment and prognosis. J Bone Joint Surg [Am] 55: 95–105
Jajić I, Rulnjević J (1979) Myositis ossificans localisata as a complication of tetanus. Acta Orthop Scand 50: 547–548

Järvi OH, Kvist HTA, Vainio PV (1968) Extraskeletal retroperitoneal osteosarcoma probably arising from myositis ossificans. Acta Pathol Microbiol Scand 74: 11–25

Johnson JTH (1957) Atypical myositis ossificans. J Bone Joint Surg [Am] 39: 189–194

Johnson MK, Lawrence JF (1975) Metaplastic bone formation (myositis ossificans) in the soft tissues of the hand. Case report. J Bone Joint Surg [Am] 57: 999–1000

Jokl P, Federico J (1977) Myositis ossificans traumatica. Association with hemophilia (factor XI deficiency) in a football player. JAMA 237: 2215–2216

Jones BV, Ward MW (1980) Myositis ossificans in the biceps femoris muscles causing sciatic nerve palsy. A case report. J Bone Joint Surg [Br] 62: 506–507

Kagan AR, Steckel RJ (1978) Diagnostic oncology case studies. Heterotopic new bone formation: Myositis ossificans versus malignant tumor. AJR 130: 773–776

Khalifa MC, Amr F, Fouly SE, Aouf M (1981) Ossification of the anterior longitudinal ligament of the spine as a cause of dysphagia. J Laryngol Otol 95: 527–528

Kleiman SG, Stevens J, Kolb L, Pankovich A (1971) Late sciatic nerve palsy following posterior fracture-dislocation of the hip. J Bone Joint Surg [Am] 53: 781–782

Kohler A (1903) Roentgenology. English translation by Turnbull A (1935), 2nd edn. Ballière Tindall Cox, London, p 188

Kromann-Andersen C, Sørensen TS, Hougaard K, Zdravkovic D, Frigaard E (1980) Ectopic bone formation following Charnley hip arthroplasty. Acta Orthop Scand 51: 633–638

Lazansky MG (1973) Complications revisited. The debit side of total hip replacement. Clin Orthop 95: 96–103

Lipscomb AB, Thomas ED, Johnston KJ (1976) Treatment of myositis ossificans traumatica in athletes. Am J Sports Med 4: 111–120

Lloyd FS, Deaver GG, Eastwood FR (1936) Safety in athletics. WB Saunders Co, Philadelphia, p 345

Lotke PA (1970) Ossification of the Achilles tendon. Report of seven cases. J Bone Joint Surg [Am] 52: 157–160

Mallory TB (1933) A group of metaplastic and neoplastic bone- and cartilage-containing tumors of soft parts. Am J Pathol 9: 765–776

Matos M, Amstutz HC, Finerman G (1975) Myositis ossificans following total hip replacement. J Bone Joint Surg [Am] 57: 137

Mattingly PC, Mowat AG (1980) HLA antigens in patients with ectopic ossification after total hip replacement. J Rheumatol 7: 582

Michelsson J-E, Granroth G, Andersson LC (1980) Myositis ossificans following forcible manipulation of the leg. A rabbit model for studying heterotopic bone formation. J Bone Joint Surg [Am] 62: 811–815

Mitra M, Sen AK, Deb HK (1976) Myositis ossificans traumatica: a complication of tetanus. Report of a case and review of the literature. J Bone Joint Surg [Am] 58: 885–886

Mollan RAB (1979) Serum alkaline phosphatase in heterotopic para-articular ossification after total hip replacement. J Bone Joint Surg [Br] 61: 432–434

Mulherin D, Schow CE (1980) Traumatic myositis ossificans after genioplasty. J Oral Surg 38: 786–789

Munster AM, Bruck HM, Johns LA, von Prince K, Kirkman EM, Remig RL (1972) Heterotopic calcification following burns: A prospective study. J Trauma 12: 1071–1074

Nollen AJG, Slooff TJJH (1973) Para-articular ossifications after total hip replacement. Acta Orthop Scand 44: 230–241

Norman A, Dorfman HD (1970) Juxtacortical circumscribed myositis ossificans: Evolution and radiographic features. Radiology 96: 301–306

Odiase VON (1975) Myositis ossificans as a complication of tetanus. J R Coll Surg Edinb 20: 384–386

Oliver P (1914) Myositis ossificans following a single trauma. JAMA 63: 1452–1455

Otto (1816) Cited by Binnie (1903) On myositis ossificans traumatica. Ann Surg 38: 423–440

Pack GT, Braund RR (1942) The development of sarcoma in myositis ossificans. Report of three cases. JAMA 119: 776–779

Painter CF (1921) A consideration of the etiologic factors in myositis ossificans traumatica. Boston Med Surg J 185: 45–52

Paus B (1951) Traumatic dislocation of the hip. Late results in 76 cases. Acta Orthop Scand 21: 99–112

Pelligrini A (1905) Ossificazione traumatica del ligamento collaterale tibiale del'articolazione del ginoccio sinistro. Clin Med 11: 433–439

Pellegrini A (1938) Ossificazione post-traumatische para-articulori. Arch Ital Chir 53: 501–563

Petersen J (1947) A case of osseous changes in patient with hemophilia. Acta Radiol 28: 323–330

Pinter J, Lenart G, Rischak G (1980) Histologic, physical and chemical investigation of myositis ossificans traumatica. Acta Orthop Scand 51: 899–902

Renier JC, Bonhomme R, Dohin M (1966) Deux cas de para-ostéo-arthropathies au cours de tétanos.

References

Rev Rhum 33: 481–486

Resnick D, Linovitz J, Feingold ML (1976) Postoperative heterotopic ossification in patients with ankylosing hyperostosis of the spine (Forestier's disease). J Rheumatol 3: 313–320

Riegler HF, Harris CM (1976) Heterotopic bone formation after total hip arthroplasty. Clin Orthop 117: 209–216

Riska EB, Michelsson JE (1979) Treatment of para-articular ossification after total hip replacement by excision and use of free fat transplants. Acta Orthop Scand 50: 751–754

Ritter MA, Vaughan RB (1977) Ectopic ossification after total hip arthroplasty. Predisposing factors, frequency and effect on result. J Bone Joint Surg [Am] 59: 345–351

Rosendahl S, Christoffersen JK, Nørgaard M (1977) Para-articular ossification following hip replacement. 70 arthroplasties ad modum Moore using McFarland's approach. Acta Orthop Scand 48: 400–404

Salvati EA, Im VC, Aglietti P, Wilson PD Jr (1976) Radiology of total hip replacements. Clin Orthop 121: 74–82

Sampinato F (1970) Ossificazioni modellate nelle parti molli in soggetti emofilici. Riv Radiol 10: 52–61

Schiele HP, Hubbard RB, Bruck HM (1972) Radiographic changes in burns of the upper extremity. Radiology 104: 13–18

Schneider RC, Papo M, Alvarez C (1962) The effects of chronic recurrent spinal trauma in high diving. A study of Acapulco's divers. J Bone Joint Surg [Am] 44: 648–656

Severi R (1933) Produzione sperimentale di cartilagine e di osso in seguito ad iniezioni di un sale di chinino. Pathologica 25: 611–619

Shanoff LB, Spira M, Hardy SB (1967) Myositis ossificans: Evolution to osteogenic sarcoma. Report of a histologically verified case. Am J Surg 113: 537–541

Shawkat AH (1967) Myositis ossificans. Report of a case. Oral Surg 23: 751–754

Slätis P, Kiviluoto O, Santavirta S (1978) Ectopic ossification after hip arthroplasty. Ann Chir Gynaecol 67: 89–93

Stauffer RN, Sim FH (1976) Total hip arthroplasty in Paget's disease of the hip. J Bone Joint Surg [Am] 58: 476–478

Stieda A (1908) Über eine typische Verletzung am unteren Femurende. Arch Klin Chir 85: 815–826

Taylor AR, Kamdar BA, Arden GP (1976) Ectopic ossification following total hip replacement. J Bone Joint Surg [Br] 58: 134

Thakkar DH, Porter RW (1981) Heterotopic ossification enveloping the sciatic nerve following posterior fracture-dislocation of the hip: A case report. Injury 13: 207–209

Thompson HC III, Garcia A (1967) Myositis ossificans: Aftermath of elbow injuries. Clin Orthop 50: 129–134

Thorndike A Jr (1940) Myositis ossificans traumatica. J Bone Joint Surg 22: 315–323

Tredget T, Godberson CV, Bose B (1977) Myositis ossificans due to hockey injury. Can Med Assoc J 116: 65–66

van der Heul RO, von Ronnen JR (1967) Juxtacortical osteosarcoma. Diagnosis, differential diagnosis and an analysis of eighty cases. J Bone Joint Surg [Am] 49: 415–439

Vas W, Cockshott WP, Martin RF, Pai NK, Walker I (1981) Myositis ossificans in hemophilia. Skeletal Radiol 7: 27–31

Wilkes LL (1976) Myositis ossificans traumatica in a young child. A case report. Clin Orthop 118: 151–152

Zadek I (1969) Ossifying hematoma in the thigh. A case report. J Bone Joint Surg [Am] 51: 386–390

3 Tumor Ossification

Ossification may occur in a wide variety of benign and malignant tumors. Ossifying tumors may arise in the skeleton, the viscera or the soft tissues and are classified according to tissue of origin and histological characteristics. Primary bone tumors, with the exception of parosteal osteosarcoma, are outside the scope of this monograph since they are unlikely to be confused with ossifying tumors of the soft tissues.

Parosteal Osteosarcoma

Parosteal osteosarcoma is characterized by an origin on the external surface of a bone and a high degree of structural differentiation. Growth is relatively slow and the prognosis is better than in the usual type of osteosarcoma of bone (WHO classification: Schajowicz et al. 1972). First recognized as a distinct entity by Geschickter and Copeland in 1951, this is an uncommon primary tumor of bone. Dahlin (1978) found only 36 cases out of 6221 primary bone tumors which had been seen in the Mayo Clinic up to 1978. Parosteal osteosarcoma thus accounts for less than 1% of all primary bone tumors and only 3%–4% of all osteosarcomas. By 1967 80 cases had been reported in the world literature (van der Heul and von Ronnen 1967). Synonyms for this tumor include: parosteal osteoma and juxtacortical osteogenic sarcoma.

Clinical Features

Typically, a young adult presents with a slow-growing mass, often of several years' duration. Almost all of the recorded cases involved the femur, humerus or tibia, although rarely other bones may be affected. Dull pain may be present and there may be some limitation of movement at an adjacent joint. The numbers of male and female patients are equal, and the average age at presentation is about 10 years older than for the usual type of osteosarcoma. In the large series of Stevens et al. (1957) the average age at diagnosis was 30 years.

Up to one-third of patients have a vague history of antecedent trauma but in general the past history is unremarkable. Examination reveals a hard mass arising from one of the long bones. Results of routine laboratory tests are usually within normal limits.

Radiology

These lesions usually arise from the long bones, especially the popliteal surface of the distal femur. Rarely, lesions occur in the foot, hand, clavicle, scapula, mastoid or mandible (Som and Peimer 1961, Stark et al. 1971). Tumors usually arise from the metaphysis of the affected bone. Typically, there is a firm cortical attachment along a part of its sessile base and the growth tends to encircle the adjacent bone with a 1 to 3 mm gap between growth and bone, the so-called string sign (Stevens et al. 1957). Oblique views or tomography may be necessary to demonstrate this gap. Computerized tomography is also useful in this respect. The tumor is usually lobular and the periphery tends to be less densely ossified than the base. Characteristic irregular radiolucent defects which correspond to areas of cartilage or fibrous tissue may be seen. Helpful and distinctive radiological features are the absence of periosteal elevation and the intact underlying cortex. Medullary involvement, if it occurs, is a late feature.

Angiography reveals no abnormal vascularity of the tumor. Adjacent major blood vessels are displaced by the mass rather than becoming encased in it: angiography may therefore be helpful in planning surgery (Probst 1971).

Pathology

This tumor is hard, lobulated and well delineated. Size varies from 3 to 25 cm in diameter with an average of 10 cm (Huvos 1979). The cut surface is greyish-white. Histopathology reveals regular osseous trabeculae, with atypical spindle-shaped or polyhedral cells between. The fact that these spaces between the trabeculae are not filled with fat or hemopoietic tissue serves to distinguish this lesion from a cartilaginous exostosis (Dahlin 1978). A variable number of fibrous and cartilaginous foci may be seen. At the periphery of the tumor admixture with muscle and fat cells is commonly observed. Evidence of malignancy may be found only in very small foci and thus histological diagnosis may be difficult in the absence of clinical and radiological information. Ahuja et al. (1977) suggest a histological grading into three types which has prognostic importance.

Pathogenesis

Parosteal osteosarcoma is believed to arise from the periosteum. Although up to one-third of patients have a vague history of antecedent trauma, the etiological significance of this is uncertain.

Natural History

Slow growth is characteristic and there is dispute whether this lesion is initially benign and only later becomes malignant (Fine and Stout 1956) or is actually a low-grade malignant process from the start (Dwinnell et al. 1954). Certainly many patients will develop metastatic disease if given inadequate therapy and so treatment has to be aggressive.

Management

Recurrence is likely after limited excision so amputation is usually required. With such therapy cure is to be expected and parosteal osteosarcoma represents the most curable primary bone tumor. In major series the reported survival rates 5 years after initial therapy were 70%–80% (Dwinnell et al. 1954, Scaglietti and Calandriello 1962, van der Heul and von Ronnen 1967, Farr and Huvos 1972, Dahlin, 1978). In Campanacci and Giunti's (1976) series the 10-year survival rate was 55%. Radiotherapy did not appear to enhance survival.

Soft Tissue Osteosarcoma

The soft tissue osteosarcoma is a highly malignant tumor which is characterized by direct formation of bone and osteoid tissue by the tumor cells (WHO classification: Schajowicz et al. 1972). Lorentzon et al. (1979) noted that 111 cases had been reported up to 1979, including several large series (Fine and Stout 1956, Allan and Soule 1971, Wurlitzer et al. 1972). This type of tumor is thus rare and represented only 1% of somatic soft tissue sarcomas recorded at the Mayo Clinic (Allan and Soule 1971). Only 4 cases were found in the Swedish cancer registry for the period 1958–1968 and this indicates a prevalence of 1 per 22 million persons (Lorentzon et al. 1979).

Clinical Features

In contrast to osteogenic sarcoma of bone, where the peak age of presentation lies between 10 and 20 years, the majority of patients with extra-osseous osteogenic sarcoma are over 30 years at diagnosis, with an average of 51 years for all of the reported cases to 1979 (Lorentzon et al. 1979). Only a few cases have been reported in childhood (Kauffman and Stout 1963). The numbers of male and female patients are equal. Forty-three of 111 cases involved the thigh and this represents the single most common site. Involvement of the soft tissues of the trunk appears to be uncommon. Patients usually notice an increasing soft tissue mass which is often painful. Characteristically this mass is hard and may be fixed to the deeper tissues. Serum alkaline phosphatase level is occasionally increased (Wurlitzer et al. 1972).

Radiology

Radiographs reveal a soft tissue mass up to 10 cm in diameter, which contains variable streaky radio-opacities. These opacities may be fuzzy and show peripheral spiculation (Fig. 3.1). The adjacent bone may be secondarily invaded, but in this case there will be a saucerized defect which indicates an external origin and aids the distinction from a primary osteosarcoma of bone which has secondarily invaded the soft tissues (Greenfield 1980).

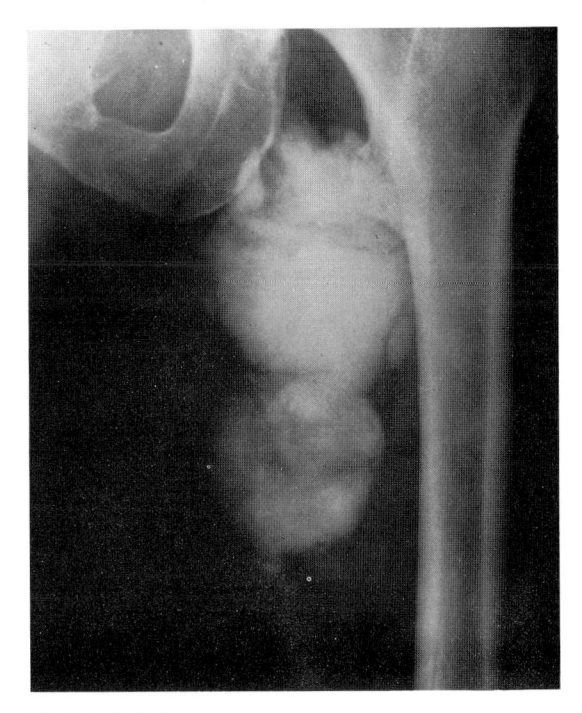

Fig.3.1. Soft tissue osteosarcoma.

Pathology

Lesions are usually poorly circumscribed although they may show pseudo-encapsulation (Ackerman 1958). In contrast to the pseudomalignant osseous tumors of soft tissue (see p. 46), no zonal phenomenon is evident and the highly cellular stroma shows features of malignancy with pleomorphism, excessive mitotic activity and abnormal mitotic figures. Osteoid is atypical and irregularly distributed and multinucleated giant cells may be seen. Central necrosis is common (Allan and Soule 1971, Rao et al. 1978).

Pathogenesis

Fine and Stout (1956) stated that 15% of cases arose in areas of post-traumatic ossification. This association has not been evident in subsequent studies and the etiological importance of trauma to these lesions is not now accepted (Allan and Soule 1971). A few reports have described an area of established post-traumatic bone undergoing neoplastic transformation (Pack and Braund 1942—case 1, Kagan and Steckel 1978), but this risk is probably no greater for ectopic bone than for the normal skeleton. Similarly, the 30-year-old patient described by Eckardt et al. (1981) who developed a soft tissue osteosarcoma in an area of soft tissue calcification secondary to childhood dermatomyositis appears to be an exceptional case.

Radiation therapy carries a small but definite increased risk of subsequent bone sarcoma (Phillips and Sheline 1963). Likewise, soft tissue osteosarcoma arising in an irradiated field has also been described in at least 4 patients (Boyer and Navin, 1965). The interval between the irradiation and the diagnosis of sarcoma ranged from 4 to 11 years. No differences were noted with respect to histology or clinical progression between these patients and those with spontaneous tumors.

Natural History

Soft tissue osteosarcoma is a highly malignant tumor which metastasizes early to the lungs.

Management

Recurrence is to be expected after local excision and this form of therapy has not produced any long-term survivors. Those with the most experience in this disease seem to agree that radical excision of the tumor *en bloc* is necessary (Allan and Soule 1971, Wurlitzer et al. 1972). Excision should include all the surrounding soft tissue and underlying muscles without disturbing the tumor mass; thus many patients will require amputation. With radical surgery Allan and Soule (1971) noted that 5 of 18 patients were alive at 5 years and the average patient survival was 3–4 years. Radiotherapy, or chemotherapy with dactinomycin, nitrogen mustard or cyclophosphamide, has not produced any objective benefit.

Other Ossifying Connective Tissue Tumors

Lipomas are the commonest soft tissue tumors (Myhre-Jensen 1981). Beck in 1858 reported a 44-year-old female who died of cachexia secondary to superficial ulceration of an ossified lipoma of her right thigh. This tumor weighed 27.5 kg and the bony mass was the size of a child's head. The few subsequent reports of ossified lipomas have been somewhat less dramatic and Tang et al. were able to find 13 well-documented examples up to 1981. Typically, they occur in the limbs, are well encapsulated and have no attachment to the underlying bone (Plaut et al. 1959). The radiological appearance is characteristic, with bone in a well-defined lucent zone (Murphy 1974). The prevalence of ossification in lipomas is unknown, but would appear to be rare. None of the 626 lipomas in the series of Myhre-Jensen (1981) contained bone.

Hemangiomas of skeletal muscle may also ossify. This was first recorded by Bishop in 1936 and has been recently reviewed by Engelstad et al. (1980). More than 90% of skeletal muscle hemangiomas are discovered before 30 years of age, the numbers of male and female patients are equal, and most hemangiomas occur in the muscles of the forearm or thigh. Most patients present with a soft tissue swelling which has grown slowly and there may be vague local pain. Elevation of the extremity or application of a tourniqet may alter the size of the swelling and phleboliths in the mass may be palpable (Jones 1953). Radiographs show phleboliths in most patients and occasionally there may be a periosteal reaction (Heitzman and Jones 1960). When present, ossification may show a characteristic Swiss cheese pattern. Surgical excision will relieve symptoms and prevent the occasional complication of pathological muscle rupture.

Ossification is a common finding in mesenchymomas (mixed mesenchymal tumors). These tumors, which may be benign or malignant, contain more than one neoplastic component of mesenchymal origin (Stout 1948). Common sites are the peri-renal and renal tissues, the mediastinum, spinal canal, liver, chest wall and extremities. Even when benign, mesenchymomas are infiltrating tumors and tend to recur after local excision. Fine and Stout (1956) noted that of 218 benign mesenchymomas which were on the the Surgical Pathology records of Columbia University up to 1954, some 53 (24%) contained bone; their equivalent figures for malignant mesenchymomas were 52 (28%) of 186.

There have been occasional case reports of ossification in other connective tissue tumors including: pseudosarcomatous soft tissue proliferation (Dahl and Angervall 1977); giant cell tumor of soft tissue (Kwittken and Branche 1969); fibromas (Gay et al. 1975, Walter et al. 1979); lipofibroma of the median nerve (Louis and Dick 1973); an ossifying limbal desmoid (Weinstein et al. 1979); and embryonal rhabdomyosarcoma (Brasch et al. 1981).

Ossifying Skin Tumors

Roth et al. (1963) assembled a large series of 120 patients with cutaneous ossification and reviewed the previously reported 305 cases in the literature. Nearly one-half of all cases of skin ossification were due to ossification in skin tumors and pilomatrixoma was the commonest single cause.

A pilomatrixoma (calcifying epithelioma of Malherbe) is believed to arise from primitive epidermal germ cells which are differentiating towards hair matrix cells. This tumor type was first described in 1880 by Malherbe and Chenantain. Forbis and Helwig (1961) surveyed the literature and found 303 reported cases to which they added 240 of their own. Clinically most lesions appear as solitary, painless nodules on the neck or arms of children or young adults (Fig. 3.2). Epidermal cysts are clinically similar except that they tend to occur on the scalp in an older age group. Histopathological features have been discussed in detail by Forbis and Helwig (1961). These authors noted calcification in 84% of pilomatrixomata and ossification in 20%. Bone occurred mainly in the periphery of the tumor. Despite this tumor's alternative name, this lesion is benign and is cured by local excision.

Hirsch and Helwig (1961) reported 188 cases of chondroid syringoma (mixed tumor of skin–salivary gland type). Patients usually had a firm subcutaneous or intracutaneous nodule which had been present for several years with little or no increase in size. Cartilage was commonly found in these tumors but bone was rare. Although usually benign, occasional malignant chondroid syringomas have been reported (Redono et al. 1982).

Bone has been described in cutaneous nevi. These have usually been intradermal nevi on the face (Meltzer 1950, Roth et al. 1963). Bone may also be occasionally found at the base of a basal cell carcinoma (Roth et al. 1963).

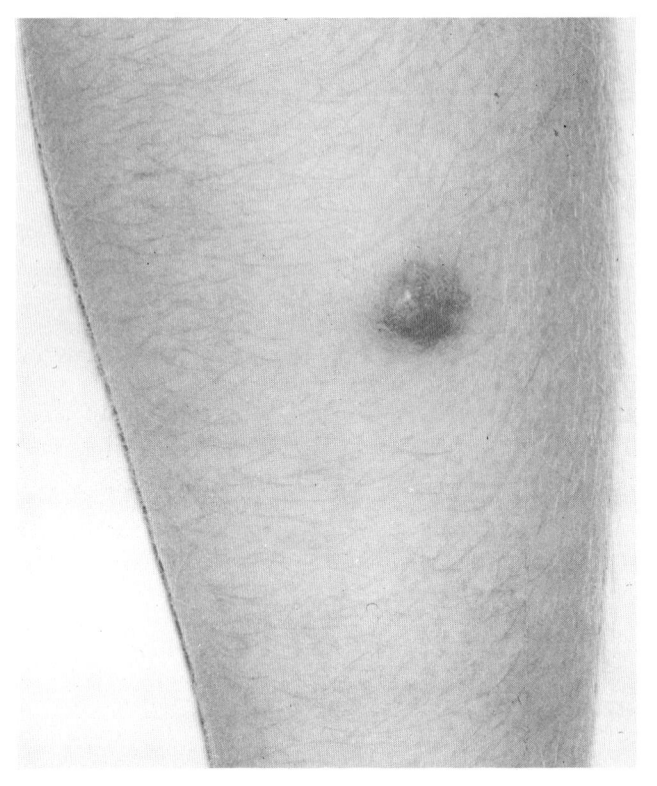

Fig. 3.2. Pilomatrixoma.

Visceral Tumor Ossification

Calcification in visceral tumors is common and has been occasionally reported in virtually all tumor types (Stein 1935, Gemell 1964, Black and Young 1965, Ferris and O'Connor 1965, Dalinka et al. 1975). Ossification is not uncommon in teratomas but is rare in other visceral tumors, with only 38 cases in the world literature up to 1968 (Kreuzer and Staffeldt 1968). This figure excludes ossification in breast tumors (see below).

Teratomas have the unique ability amongst tumors to differentiate in the direction of all three germ layers. By definition, teratomas are present at birth, although they often do not manifest until later life. In childhood most are found in the sacrococcygeal region (Fig. 3.3), the next most common site being the gonads (Mahour et al. 1974). In adults, the testes, ovaries and mediastinum are the most frequent sites. Occasional cases occur in brain, orbit, anterior neck, nasopharynx, stomach or retroperitoneal tissues (Berry et al. 1969).

Fine and Stout (1956) noted that up to 1956 there had been 72 case reports of osteosarcoma arising in the viscera; however, they went on to suggest that some if not all of these represented malignant growth of a single component in a teratoma. Not all would agree with this and certainly osteosarcoma of the breast would appear to be a distinct tumor type, with 116 reported cases up to 1963 (Jernstrom

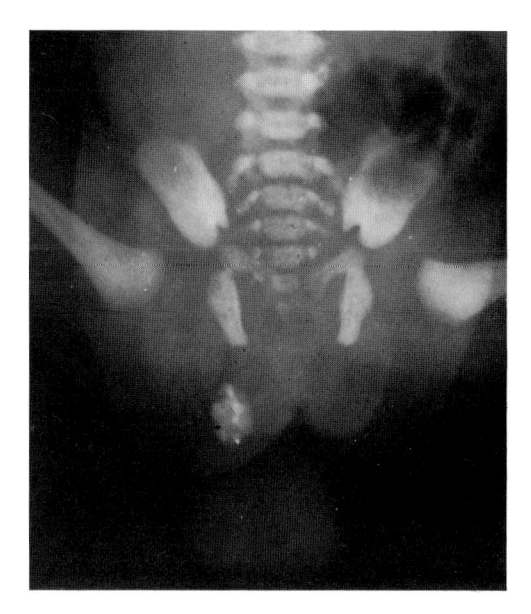

Fig.3.3. Sacrococcygeal teratoma in a neonate.

et al. 1963). The first case of a malignant mammary tumor which contained bone was reported by Bonet in 1700 and succeeding cases have been reported under a wide variety of names including: teratoid mixed tumor (McIver 1923), osteoid sarcoma (Rottino and Howley 1945) and osteochondrofibrosarcoma (Carlucci and Wagner 1943).

Breast tumors containing bone have usually been histologically classified as sarcomas. Breast sarcomas account for 0.9%–3% of all breast malignancies and 5%–12.8% of these sarcomas contain bone (Sun 1952). Patients are usually middle-aged or elderly, with a lobulated occasionally cystic mass in the breast which may be mobile or fixed. Metastasis is hematogenous rather than lymphatic to regional nodes. Radical surgery offers the only prospect of cure, but despite surgery the prognosis remains poor (Cole-Beuglet et al. 1976).

Ossification of tumors of the gastrointestinal tract has been mostly found in colorectal adenocarcinomas. Dukes (1938), on the basis of his extensive experience with these tumors, estimated that ossification occurred in up to 0.4% of rectal malignancies. In the three cases described by Christie (1951), intramembranous ossification occurred in close proximity to living neoplastic epithelium. Bone has also been recorded in tumors of the appendix and stomach (Rhone and Horowitz 1976).

Ossification, although rare in squamous cell carcinomas of the bronchus, is present in up to 16% of all bronchial adenomas and up to 30% of bronchial carcinoid tumors (Flanagan et al. 1965, Kinney and Kovarick 1965, Cooney et al. 1979). In the case of carcinoid tumors bone forms in bronchial cartilage which is contiguous with, or has been engulfed by, the tumor. The amount of bone in these tumors is rarely sufficient to show on a chest radiograph but may be apparent on computerized tomography (Cooney et al. 1979).

Pang (1958) reported 5 new and reviewed 15 previously reported cases of ossification in the stroma of transitional cell carcinomas of the bladder.

Osteogenic sarcoma of bone may metastasize to viscera or soft tissues and then produce bone at these distant sites (Goldstein et al. 1977).

Less commonly, a visceral tumor may produce heterotopic bone-forming metastases. This has been reported from colorectal adenocarcinoma (Senturia et al. 1948, van Patter and Whittick 1955, Engel and Dockerty 1962, Govoni and Alcantara 1968), carcinoma of the stomach (Yasuma et al. 1973), carcinoma of the breast (Patel and Maso 1966), follicular carcinoma of the thyroid (Wasiljew et al. 1981) and transitional cell carcinoma of the urinary epithelium (Cornes et al. 1960, Briggs and Wegner 1966, Chinn et al. 1976). Ossification in these metastases may occur without corresponding ossification in the primary tumor (Laubman 1932, Cornes et al. 1960, Lisbona et al. 1972, Rhone and Horowitz 1976, Evison et al. 1981). This suggests that the bone is being produced by local connective tissue cells, rather than by metaplasia of tumor cells to osteoblasts. In this respect, an enlightening case was described by Bettendorf et al. (1976) of metastatic adenocarcinoma of the bronchus. Extensive bone occurred in the metastases but not the primary tumor. Further, ossification only occurred in close anatomical proximity to the cancer tissue and was restricted to metastases within skeletal muscles and in the neighborhood of tendons and ligaments. The size of the metastasis was also important: small metastases failed to ossify and ossification was absent at the center of large lesions.

The development of ossification within visceral tumors or their metastases is thus rare. With **metastatic deposits**, as illustrated by the above cases, the tumors seem to activate local mesenchymal cells, presumably the inducible osteogenic precursor cells (see p. 112), to become osteoblasts. Similarly, in ossifying primary tumors, activation of local mesenchyme may be more important than differentiation of tumor cells into osteoblasts. Teratomas are the exception to this, since by definition they have the ability to differentiate into derivatives of any germ layer.

If visceral tumors usually produce bone by local activation of mesenchymal cells, then why does this only occur in a small percentage of patients with tumors? Presumably not all tumors have the ability to activate the mesenchymal cells or perhaps normally there is a mechanism to prevent such mesenchymal transformation. In this respect, Scheidegger (1939) reported a patient who had ossification in three separate primary neoplasms: a rectal adenocarcinoma, a small mammary fibroadenoma and a leiomyoma of the stomach. Thus there may be an individual propensity towards this complication of neoplasia.

Pseudomalignant Myositis Ossificans

Although not neoplastic, pseudomalignant myositic ossificans is included in this chapter as it is commonly confused with ossifying soft tissue neoplasms. Pseudomalignant myositis ossificans was first distinguished as a separate entity by Fine and Stout in 1956. Ogilvie-Harris and Fornasier (1980) found 83 cases in the world literature up to 1980 and added a further 26 cases.

As with many conditions of unknown etiology, a variety of names have been used for this condition: pseudomalignant osseous tumor of soft tissue (Fine and Stout 1956, Jeffreys and Stiles 1966); myositis ossificans circumscripta (Paterson 1970); non-traumatic myositis ossificans in healthy individuals; and pseudomalignant myositis ossificans (Lagier and Cox 1975). None of these names has gained universal acceptance and the reader is further cautioned that some, such as myositis ossificans circumscripta, have also been used in the past to refer to post-traumatic ossification in muscles.

Clinical Features

Most patients are less than 30 years of age at presentation; peak incidence is in the second decade and there is a slight predominance of males. A painful expanding soft tissue mass is noticed, occasionally with overlying erythema. Pain tends to be maximal for the first 2–3 weeks and stops after 8 weeks when the lesion stops growing (Ogilvie-Harris and Fornasier 1980). Any muscle may be involved but there are a number of characteristic sites: adjacent to the anterior superior iliac spine, at the superior lip of the acetabulum, at the greater trochanter, at the linea aspera in the mid-part of the femur, at the mid-part of the humeral shaft, and adjacent to the first and second metacarpals. Lesions are uncommon in the vicinity of the knee and no lesions have been described in the forearms or about the elbows. Routine hematological and biochemical values are within normal limits (Paterson 1970).

Radiology

Two to three weeks after the onset of pain and swelling, flocculent radio-opacities can be seen. The mass remains circumscribed and becomes characteristically more dense peripherally. Demonstration of this central radiolucent zone, if necessary by tomography, is an important aid in diagnosis. A further helpful point is the separation of the mass from the underlying cortex by a radiolucent line. Occasional patients have a periosteal reaction, which may precede opacification of the soft tissue mass, and in these cases it may be difficult to demonstrate this radiolucent line. Over 4–6 weeks ossification increases and the lesion becomes more evenly radio-opaque (Figs. 3.4 and 3.5). Other helpful radiological features are the diaphyseal location, and the loss of volume on serial films (Goldman 1976).

Angiography is useful in the differential diagnosis from a soft tissue neoplasm. In the early stages, numerous fine blood vessels are present which produce a diffuse blush. Later the lesion is avascular or nearly so. There are never the pathological blood vessels, amputated blood vessels, arteriovenous shunting and venous lakes that may be seen with malignant soft tissue tumors (Yaghmai 1977). Bone scan reveals an isolated, well-demarcated area of uptake. The ultrasound appearance of a soft tissue mass with a central echogenicity due to calcification is not specific for this disorder (Kramer et al. 1979).

Pathology

A characteristic zoning pattern of peripheral maturation is present. This was first stressed by Ackerman (1958) and has been a consistent feature in subsequent reports. The lesions are 1–6 cm in diameter and are easily separated at operation from the surrounding soft tissues. They appear white and glistening on cut section. The central zone consists of undifferentiated mesenchymal cells with plentiful, but normal, mitotic figures and occasional giant cells. This is surrounded by an

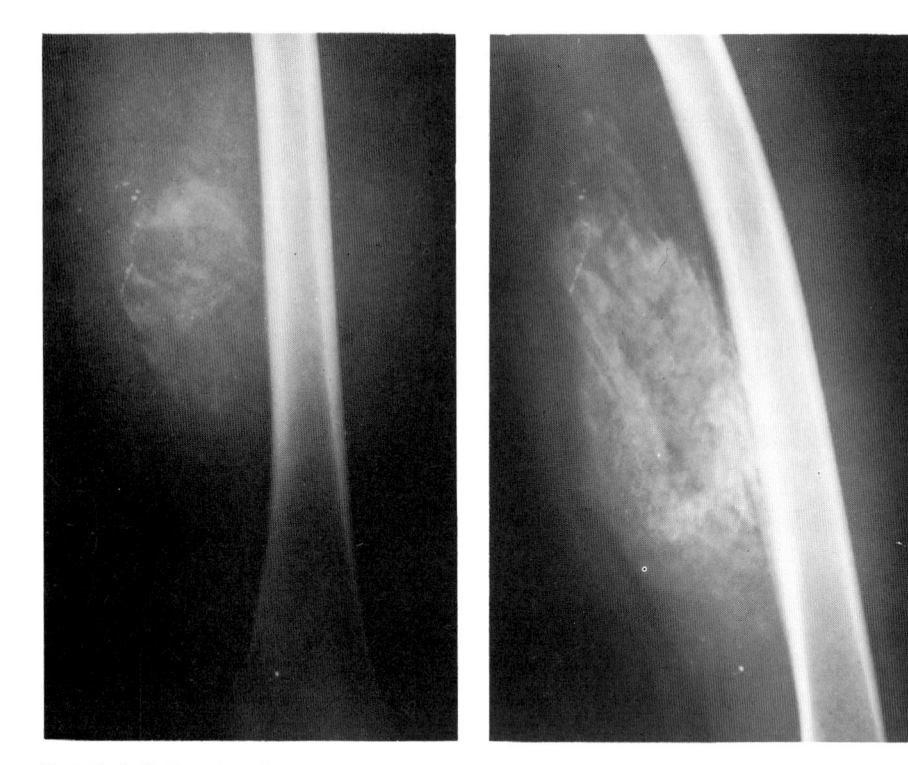

Fig.3.4. (*left*) Pseudomalignant myositis ossificans 3 weeks from onset.
Fig.3.5. (*right*) Pseudomalignant myositis ossificans 6 weeks from onset (same patient as Fig. 3.4).

intermediate zone which contains osteoid and finally there is a zone of maturing bone (Figs. 3.6 and 3.7). There is no evidence of invasion of surrounding tissues. Intact muscle fibers may be found in all three zones of these lesions: this is diagnostically useful as it would be most unusual in a malignant tumor. By 6–8 weeks the lesion consists of uniform mature bone. The diagnostic histological appearance may not be readily apparent on a needle biopsy and on the basis of the central tissue only from a lesion a misdiagnosis of a malignancy may be made. It is important to note that the characteristic zoning may be poorly established in a biopsy during the first week.

Pathogenesis

These lesions represent focal mesenchymal proliferations but the stimulus for this proliferation is obscure. There is no clear relationship with previous trauma. The occurrence is sporadic with no reports of similarly affected family members.

Natural History

The majority of these lesions are excised and so the untreated natural history is based on relatively few cases. Ogilvie-Harris and Fornasier (1980) described 2

Pseudomalignant Myositis Ossificans

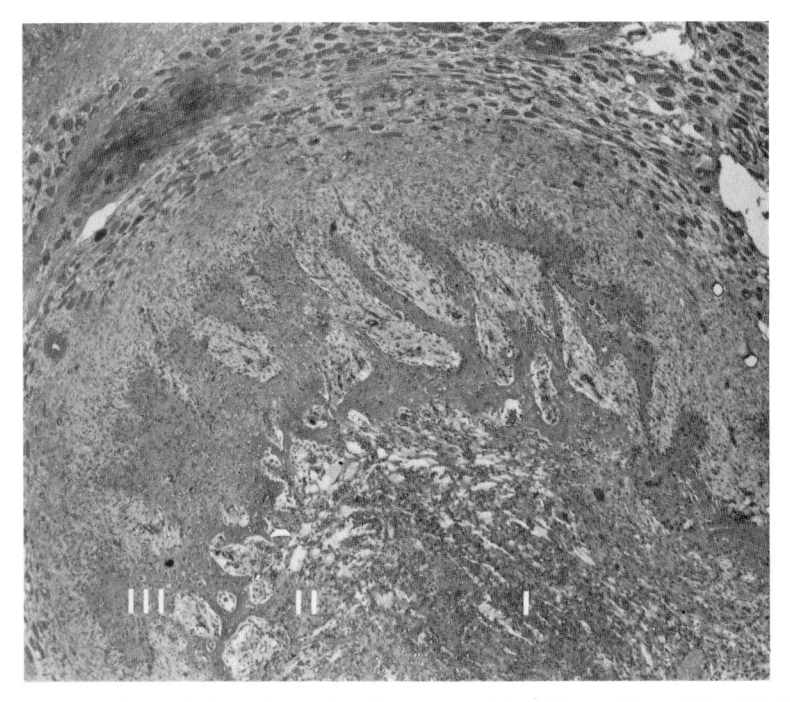

Fig.3.6. Histopathology of pseudomalignant myositis ossificans (H and E, ×25). Inner zone I of proliferating mesenchyme; zone II of osteoid; and zone III of maturing bone.

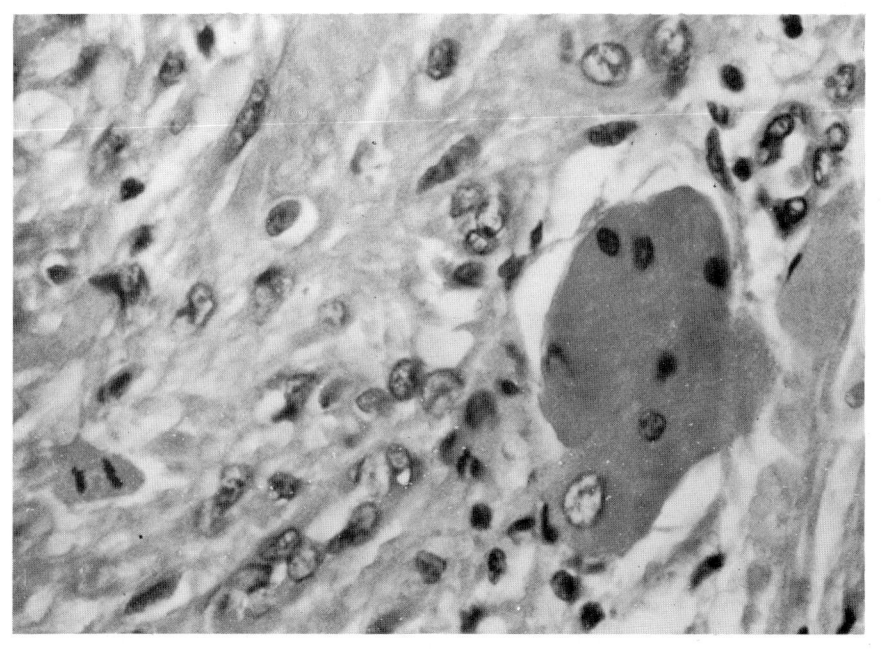

Fig.3.7. Histopathology of inner zone in pseudomalignant myositis ossificans (H and E, ×500).

patients who were conservatively treated. Both were young boys; in one the lesion spontaneously resolved over 3 years, in the other it was still present at 5 years although it did not increase in size after the first 8 weeks. Chaplin and Harrison (1972) described a 15-year-old girl with a lesion in her thigh which became asymptomatic, shrank, and became densely ossified over an 18-month period.

All authors stress the benign nature of this condition; local invasion or distant metastasis are not features of pseudomalignant myositis ossificans.

An affected patient does not appear to be at risk for future ossification at other sites.

Management

Excision is indicated for histological diagnosis and for the relief of mechanical obstruction or pain.

References

Ackerman LV (1958) Extra-osseous localized non-neoplastic bone and cartilage formation (so-called myositis ossificans). Clinical and pathological confusion with malignant neoplasm. J Bone Joint Surg [Am] 40: 279–298

Ahuja SC, Villacin AB, Smith J, Bullough PG, Huvos AG, Marcove RC (1977) Juxtacortical (parosteal) osteogenic sarcoma. Histological grading and prognosis. J Bone Joint Surg [Am] 59: 632–647

Allan CJ, Soule EH (1971) Osteogenic sarcoma of the somatic soft tissues. Clinicopathologic study of 26 cases and review of the literature. Cancer 27: 1121–1133

Beck B (1858) Ein Fall von ungewöhnlicher Knocken-Neubildung in einer 55 Pfunde schweren Faser-Fettgeschwulst. Arch Pathol Anat 15: 153–158

Berry CL, Keeling J, Hilton C (1969) Teratomata in infancy and childhood: A review of 91 cases. J Pathol 98: 241–252

Bettendorf U, Remmele W, Laaff H (1976) Bone formation by cancer metastases: Case report and review of the literature. Virchows Arch 369: 359–365

Bishop BWF (1936) Haemangioma of voluntary muscle. Br J Surg 24: 190–191

Black JW, Young B (1965) A radiological and pathological study of the incidence of calcification in diseases of the breast and neoplasms of other tissues. Br J Radiol 38: 596–598

Bonet T (1700) Mammae osseae in virgine cum pectoris hydrope, in sepulchretum sine anatomia practica ex-cadaveribus morbo denatis, vol 2. Cramer and Perachon, Geneva, p 522

Boyer CW Jr, Navin JJ (1965) Extraskeletal osteogenic sarcoma: a late complication of radiation therapy. Cancer 18: 628–633

Brasch RC, Kim OH, Kushner JH, Rosenau W (1981) Ossification in a soft tissue embryonal rhabdomyosarcoma. Pediatr Radiol 11: 99–101

Briggs RC, Wegner GP (1966) Osseous metaplasia in soft tissue. Demonstration of metastasis by Sr^{85} scintiscanning. JAMA 195: 1061–1064

Campanacci M, Giunti A (1976) Parosteal osteosarcoma. Review of 41 cases, 22 with long-term follow-up. Ital J Orthop 1: 23–25

Carlucci GA, Wagner RF (1943) Osteochondrofibrosarcoma of the breast. Case report. Am J Surg 61: 271–276

Chaplin DM, Harrison MHM (1972) Pseudomalignant osseous tumor of soft tissue. J Bone Joint Surg [Br] 54: 334–340

Chinn D, Genant HK, Quivey JM, Carlsson A-M (1976) Heterotopic-bone formation in metastatic tumor from transitional-cell carcinoma of the urinary bladder. J Bone Joint Surg [Am] 58: 881–883

Christie AC (1951) Ossification in intestinal neoplasms: A report of three cases. J Pathol Bacteriol 63: 338–343

References

Cole-Beuglet C, Kirk ME, Selouan R, Arzoumanian A, Brown RA (1976) Bone within the breast. Report of a case with radiographic and nuclear medicine features. Radiology 119: 643–644
Cooney T, Sweeney EC, Luke D (1979) Pulmonary carcinoid tumors: A comparative regional study. J Clin Pathol 32: 1100–1109
Cornes JS, Sussman T, Dawson IM (1960) Bone formation in metastasis from carcinoma of urinary bladder: Report of a case with review of the literature. Br J Urol 32: 290–294
Dahl I, Angervall L (1977) Pseudosarcomatous proliferative lesions of soft tissue with or without bone formations. Acta Pathol Microbiol Scand 85: 577–589
Dahlin DC (1978) Bone tumors, 3rd edn. Charles C Thomas, Springfield, Illinois
Dalinka MK, Lally JF, Azimi F, Gingerilli F (1975) Calcification in undifferentiated abdominal malignancies. Clin Radiol 26: 115–119
Dukes CE (1938) Ossification in rectal cancer. Proc R Soc Med 32: 1489–1494
Dwinnell LA, Dahlin DC, Ghormley RK (1954) Parosteal (juxtacortical) osteogenic sarcoma. J Bone Joint Surg [Am] 36: 732–744
Eckardt JJ, Ivins JC, Perry HO, Unni KK (1981) Osteosarcoma arising in heterotopic ossification of dermatomyositis: Case report and review of the literature. Cancer 48: 1256–1261
Engel S, Dockerty MB (1962) Calcification and ossification in rectal malignant processes. JAMA 179: 347–350
Engelstad BL, Gilula LA, Kyriakos M (1980) Ossified skeletal muscle hemangioma: Radiologic and pathologic features. Skeletal Radiol 5: 35–40
Evison G, Pizey N, Roylance J (1981) Bone formation associated with osseous metastases from bladder carcinoma. Clin Radiol 32: 303–309
Farr GH, Huvos AG (1972) Juxtacortical osteogenic sarcoma. An analysis of fourteen cases. J Bone Joint Surg [Am] 54: 1205–1216
Ferris EJ, O'Connor SJ (1965) Calcification in urinary bladder tumors. AJR 95: 447–449
Fine G, Stout AP (1956) Osteogenic sarcoma of the extraskeletal soft tissues. Cancer 9: 1027–1043
Flanagan P, McCracken AW, Cross RMcP (1965) Squamous carcinoma of the lung with osteocartilaginous stroma. J Clin Pathol 18: 403–407
Forbis R Jr, Helwig EB (1961) Pilomatrixoma (calcifying epithelioma). Arch Dermatol 83: 608–618
Gay I, Sela J, Ulmansky M, Odont D, Soskolne WA (1975) Ossifying fibroma: Report of a case. J Oral Surg 33: 368–371
Gemell NI (1964) Calcification within a gastric carcinoma: A case report. AJR 91: 779–783
Geschickter CF, Copeland MM (1951) Parosteal osteoma of bone: A new entity. Ann Surg 133: 790–806
Goldman AB (1976) Myositis ossificans circumscripta: A benign lesion with a malignant differential diagnosis. AJR 126: 32–40
Goldstein C, Ambos MA, Bosniak MA (1977) Multiple ossified metastases to the kidney from osteogenic sarcoma. AJR 128: 148–149
Govoni AF, Alcantara AN (1968) Ossifying metastatic carcinoma of the colon. AJR 104: 561–565
Greenfield GB (1980) Radiology of bone diseases, 3rd edn. JB Lippincott Co, Philadelphia Toronto
Heitzman ER Jr, Jones JB (1960) Roentgen characteristics of cavernous hemangioma of striated muscle. Radiology 74: 420–427
Hirsch P, Helwig EB (1961) Chondroid syringoma: Mixed tumor of skin, salivary gland type. Arch Dermatol 84: 835–847
Huvos AG (1979) Bone tumors. Diagnosis, treatment and prognosis. WB Saunders Co, Philadelphia London Toronto, pp 94–106
Jeffreys TE, Stiles PJ (1966) Pseudomalignant osseous tumor of soft tissue. J Bone Joint Surg [Br] 48: 488–492
Jernstrom P, Lindberg AL, Meland ON (1963) Osteogenic sarcoma of the mammary gland. Am J Clin Pathol 40: 521–526
Jones KG (1953) Cavernous hemangioma of striated muscle: A review of the literature and a report of four cases. J Bone Joint Surg [Am] 35: 717–728
Kagan AR, Steckel RJ (1978) Diagnostic oncology case studies. Heterotopic new bone formation: Myositis ossificans versus malignant tumor. AJR 130: 773–776
Kauffman SL, Stout AP (1963) Extraskeletal osteogenic sarcomas and chondrosarcomas in children. Cancer 16: 432–439
Kinney FJ, Kovarik JL (1965) Bone formation in bronchial adenoma. Am J Clin Pathol 44: 52–56
Kramer FL, Kurtz AB, Rubin C, Goldberg BB (1979) Ultrasound appearance of myositis ossificans. Skeletal Radiol 4: 19–20
Kreuzer G, Staffeldt K (1968) Über Knochenbildung in Karzinomen der weiblichen Genitaltraktes. Zentralbl Gynaekol 90: 1241–1247

Kwittken J, Branche M (1969) Fasciitis ossificans. Am J Clin Pathol 51: 251–255
Lagier R, Cox JN (1975) Pseudomalignant myositis ossificans. A pathological study of eight cases. Hum Pathol 6: 653–665
Laubman W (1932) Beitrag zur osteoplastischen Carcinose. Arch Pathol Anat 285: 169–181
Lisbona A, McLoud T, Kapusta M, Palayew MJ (1972) An unusual case of psoas muscle ossification due to metastatic carcinoma. J Can Assoc Radiol 23: 221–223
Lorentzon R, Larsson SE, Boquist L (1979) Extraosseous osteosarcoma. J Bone Joint Surg [Br] 61: 205–208
Louis DS, Dick HM (1973) Ossifying lipofibroma of the median nerve. J Bone Joint Surg [Am] 55: 1082–1084
McIver MA (1923) Teratoid mixed tumors of the breast. Report of a case. Ann Surg 77: 354–357
Mahour GH, Woolley MM, Trivedi SN, Landing BH (1974) Teratomas in infancy and childhood: Experience with 81 cases. Surgery 76: 309–318
Malherbe A, Chenantain J (1880) Note sur l'epitheliome calcifé des glandes sebacées. Prog Med Paris 8: 826–828
Meltzer L (1950) Heterotopic bone in a pigmented nevus. Arch Dermatol Syph 62: 696–697
Murphy NB (1974) Ossifying lipoma. Br J Radiol 47: 97–98
Myhre–Jensen O (1981) A consecutive 7-year series of 1331 benign soft tissue tumors. Clinicopathologic data. Comparison with sarcomas. Acta Orthop Scand 52: 287–293
Ogilvie-Harris DJ, Fornasier VL (1980) Pseudomalignant myositis ossificans: Heterotopic new bone formation without history of trauma. J Bone Joint Surg [Am] 62: 1274–1283
Pack GT, Braund RR (1942) The development of sarcoma in myositis ossificans. Report of three cases. JAMA 119: 776–779
Pang LS-C (1958) Bony and cartilaginous tumors of the urinary bladder. J Pathol Bacteriol 76: 357–377
Patel S, Maso CJ (1966) Ossification in metastases from carcinoma of the breast. JAMA 198: 1309–1311
Paterson DC (1970) Myositis ossificans circumscripta. Report of four cases without history of trauma. J Bone Joint Surg [Br] 52: 296–301
Phillips TL, Sheline GE (1963) Bone sarcomas following radiation therapy. Radiology 81: 992–996
Plaut GS, Salm R, Truscott DE (1959) Three cases of ossifying lipoma. J Pathol Bacteriol 78: 292–295
Probst FR (1971) Angiography in juxtacortical osteosarcomas. Case report with special reference to differential diagnosis. Acta Radiol 11: 49–56
Rao U, Cheng A, Didolkar MS (1978) Extraosseous osteogenic sarcoma. Clinicopathologic study of eight cases and review of literature. Cancer 41: 1488–1496
Redono C, Rocamora A, Villoria F, Garcia M (1982) Malignant mixed tumor of the skin: Malignant chondroid syringoma. Cancer 49: 1690–1696
Rhone DP, Horowitz RN (1976) Heterotopic ossification in the pulmonary metastases of gastric adenocarcinoma: Report of a case and review of the literature. Cancer 38: 1773–1780
Roth SI, Stowell RE, Helwig EB (1963) Cutaneous ossification. Report of 120 cases and review of the literature. Arch Pathol 76: 44–54
Rottino A, Howley CP (1945) Osteoid sarcoma of the breast: A complication of fibroadenoma. Arch Pathol 40: 44–50
Scaglietti O, Calandriello B (1962) Ossifying parosteal sarcoma. Parosteal osteoma or juxtacortical osteogenic sarcoma? J Bone Joint Surg [Am] 44: 635–647
Schajowicz F, Ackerman LV, Sissons HA (1972) Histological typing of bone tumors. World Health Organization, Geneva (International histological classification of tumors, No. 6.)
Scheidegger S (1939) Heterotope Knochenbildung (Beitrag zur Frage der Metaplasie). Schweiz Z Allg Pathol Bakteriol 2: 153–174
Senturia HR, Schechter SE, Hulbert B (1948) Heterotopic ossification in an area of metastasis from rectal carcinoma. AJR 60: 507–510
Som M, Peimer R (1961) Juxtacortical osteogenic sarcoma of the mandible. Arch Otolaryngol 74: 532–536
Stark HH, Jones FE, Jernstrom P (1971) Parosteal osteogenic sarcoma of a metacarpal bone. A case report. J Bone Joint Surg [Am] 53: 147–153
Stein IF (1935) Myofibroma of the ovary with heteroplastic bone formation. Am J Obstet Gynecol 30: 289–290
Stevens GM, Pugh DG, Dahlin DC (1957) Roentgenographic recognition and differentiation of parosteal osteogenic sarcoma. AJR 78: 1–12
Stout AP (1948) Mesenchymoma. The mixed tumor of mesenchymal derivatives. Ann Surg 127: 278–290
Sun PY (1952) Osteogenic sarcoma of the breast. Review of literature and report of a case. Chinese

References

Med J 70: 46–53

Tang TT, Chamoy L, Meyers A, Babbitt DP, McCreadie SR (1981) Congenital lipoma with ossification in the hand of a child. J Pediatr Surg 16: 511–514

van der Heul RO, von Ronnen JR (1967) Juxtacortical osteosarcoma. Diagnosis, differential diagnosis, treatment and an analysis of eighty cases. J Bone Joint Surg [Am] 49: 415–439

van Patter HT, Whittick JW (1955) Heterotopic ossification in intestinal neoplasms. Am J Pathol 31: 73–91

Walter JM Jr, Terry BC, Small EW, Matteson SR, Howell RM (1979) Aggressive ossifying fibroma of the maxilla: Review of the literature and report of case. J Oral Surg 37: 276–286

Wasiljew BK, Apostol JV, Rao MS (1981) Heterotopic ossification in a lymph node with metastatic follicular carcinoma of the thyroid: A case report. J Surg Oncol 17: 45–48

Weinstein JM, Romano PE, O'Grady RB (1979) Bone formation in association with a limbal dermoid. Arch Ophthalmol 97: 1121–1122

Wurlitzer F, Ayala A, Romsdahl M (1972) Extraosseous osteogenic sarcoma. Arch Surg 105: 691–695

Yaghmai I (1977) Myositis ossificans: diagnostic value of arteriography. AJR 128: 811–816

Yasuma T, Hashimoto K, Miyazawa R, Hiyama Y (1973) Bone formation and calcification in gastric cancer—case report and review of the literature. Acta Pathol Jpn 23: 155–172

4 Fibrodysplasia Ossificans Progressiva

Fibrodysplasia ossificans progressiva is a rare, inherited disorder of connective tissue in which physical handicap due to progressive soft tissue ossification accompanies characteristic skeletal malformations.

Many names have been proposed for this disease. Von Dusch first suggested myositis ossificans progressiva in 1868 and this name has been widely used in the older literature. The possessive eponym, Münchmeyer's disease, is not appropriate as he neither had the disease himself nor described the first case in the literature. Münchmeyer (1869) was, though, the first author clearly to distinguish this disorder from multiple cartilaginous exostoses.

As the body of scientific opinion began to favour a primary disorder of connective tissue, with only secondary involvement of muscle fibers, a number of new names were proposed: hyperplasia fascialis ossificans progressiva (Goto 1913), fibrocellulitis ossificans progressiva (Rosenstirn 1918), fibrositis ossificans progressiva (Greig 1931), myositis fibrosa generalisata (Stewart and MacGregor 1951) and fibrodysplasia ossificans progressiva (Bauer and Bode 1940). From this wide choice, the term fibrodysplasia ossificans progressiva, abbreviated to FOP, has now gained general acceptance and will be used in this monograph.

A patient with FOP usually develops extensive ectopic ossification and thus becomes a literal pillar of bone. One could speculate that Lot's wife, who turned into a pillar of salt, or the ancient Greeks who turned into stone after looking into the face of one of the Gorgon sisters might in fact have had FOP. However, the earliest recognized description is credited to Guy Patin (1692) who in 1648 wrote about a woman 'qui est devenue dure comme du bois'. John Freke, a surgeon at St. Bartholomew's Hospital, followed this with a more complete description in 1736:

> Yesterday there came a Boy of healthy Look, and about Fourteen Years old, to ask of us at the Hospital, what should be done to cure him of many large swellings on his Back which began about Three Years since, and have continued to grow as large on many Parts as a Penny-loaf, particularly on the Left Side: They arise from all the Vertebrae of the Neck, and reach down to the Os Sacrum; they likewise arise from every Rib of his Body, and joining together in all Parts of his Back, as the Ramifications of Coral do, they make, as it were, a fixed bony Pair of Bodice.

These two case reports represent the earliest recorded patients with any form of soft tissue ossification.

Similar case descriptions followed, but it was not until 1879 that Helferich pointed out the characteristic associated anomaly of the big toe. Gerber (1875) had previously noted deformed big toes in his patient with FOP, but had not realized the association. By 1918 Rosenstirn was able to find 115 definite cases of

FOP in the world literature. This number had risen to 470 by 1976 (Suzuki et al. 1976) and now exceeds 550. Several authors have provided comprehensive reviews of the literature (Rosenstirn 1918, MacKinnon 1924, Mair 1932, Fairbank 1950, Lutwak 1964, Tünte et al. 1967).

Most of the voluminous literature on FOP consists of single case reports, and few authors have had personal experience with 3 or more patients (Riley and Christie 1951, Lutwak 1964, McKusick 1972, Geho and Whiteside 1973, Smith et al. 1976, Rogers and Geho 1979, Hall and Sutcliffe 1979, Schroeder and Zasloff 1980). Tünte et al. (1967) studied 23 German patients with FOP and more recently Connor and Evans (1982a) identified 44 patients in the UK and studied 34 of these.

Prevalence

In 1979 a national survey was conducted in the UK which aimed to identify all patients with FOP (Connor and Evans 1982b). Forty-four definite patients were identified and their geographical distribution, according to place of birth, is indicated in Fig. 4.1. In mid-1978, 30 of these FOP patients were known to be alive in England and Wales out of a total estimated population of 49 117 300 (OPCS Monitor 1979). This indicates a minimum point prevalence of 1 patient per 1.64 million of the population at that time. If this prevalence figure is applicable to other countries, then at present there should be about 150 patients with FOP in the USA, and about 2500 in the world.

The sex ratio in early series showed a preponderance of males, but the numbers of male and female patients are now equal.

The disease was initially thought to be confined to the Anglo-Saxon race (Mather 1931, Ryan 1945), until Grewal and Das (1953) reported a typical case from India. FOP has since been reported in most ethnic groups (Lins and Abath 1959, Logacev 1964, Ebrahim et al. 1966). It has also been described in a number of animal species: pigs (Seibold and Davis 1967); a horse and a setter dog (Rosenstirn 1918); and even a sabre-toothed tiger from the Pleistocene (Moodie 1927).

Clinical Features

The principal clinical features are skeletal malformations and soft tissue ossification. Although malformations may be demonstrated radiologically at a number of sites in the skeleton, they are only evident clinically in the hands and feet. Characteristically, the big toes are short and lack a skin crease, since they each possess only a single phalanx which may be deviated laterally (Fig. 4.2). This classic appearance was evident in 27 of 34 (79%) patients in the UK series (Connor and Evans, 1982a). Less commonly, the big toes are of normal length, but are stiff from early childhood, or occasionally severe reduction defects of all toes are

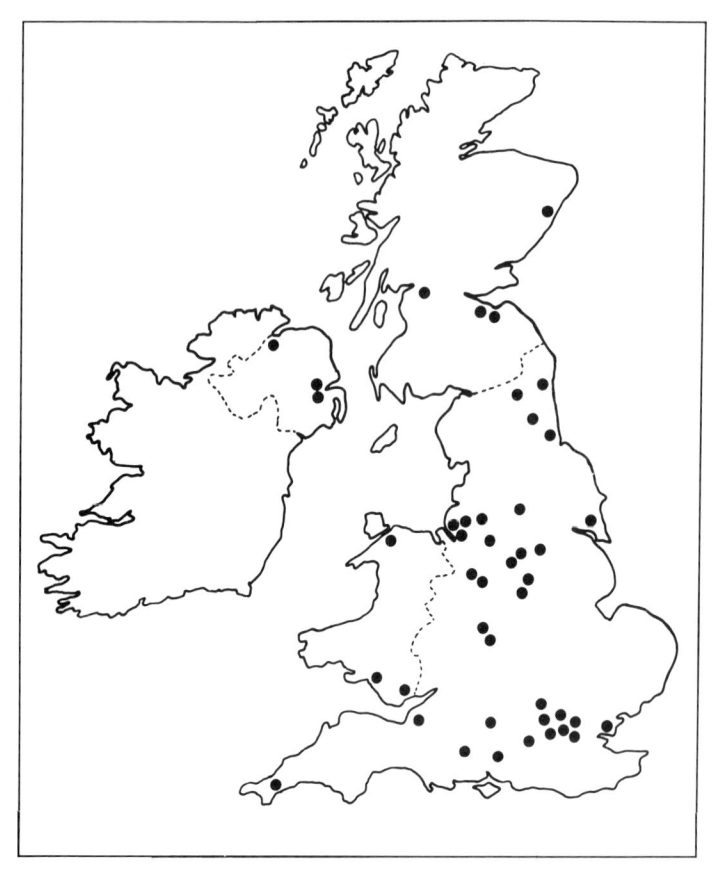

Fig. 4.1. Geographical distribution of UK patients with fibrodysplasia ossificans progressiva according to place of birth. (Reproduced with permission of the Editor, *Journal of Medical Genetics*, from Connor and Evans 1982b.)

present. Two patients in the UK series had normal big toes in early childhood on both clinical and radiological examination but developed hallux rigidus in adolescence.

Rosenstirn (1918) initially proposed the belief that abnormal big toes were present in practically all genuine cases of FOP. This view is supported by the author and by others (Tünte et al. 1967, Schroeder and Zasloff 1980) who have based their conclusions on personally evaluated series of FOP patients. The oft-quoted incidence of big toe malformations of 70%–75% has been based on retrospective surveys of the literature and no doubt reflects the incidence of the commonest, and best known, type of big toe malformation in FOP. Any of the types of big toe malformation as described above will support the diagnosis of FOP: indeed the presence of monophalangic big toes may even be pathognomonic (Schroeder and Zasloff 1980). Conversely, as occasional patients with FOP initially have normal big toes, the diagnosis is not excluded by a normal foot radiograph in early childhood and evidence of skeletal malformations at other sites should be sought.

Clinical Features

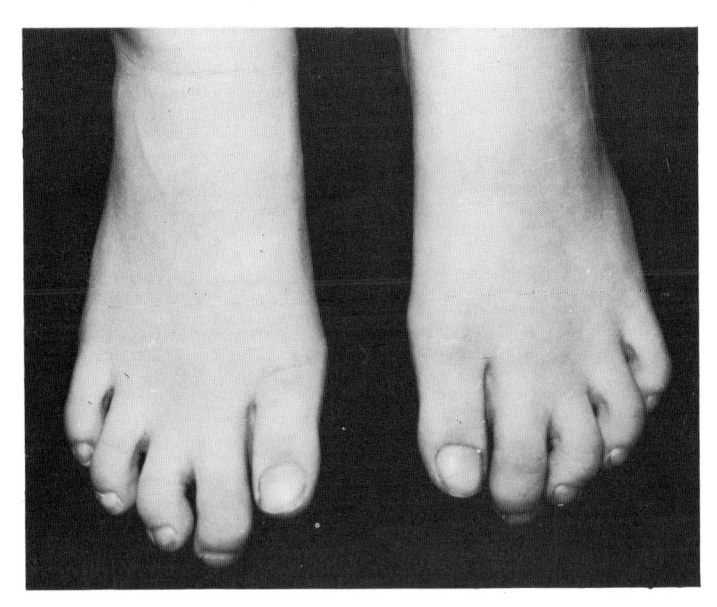

Fig. 4.2. Short big toes without valgus deviation. (Reproduced with permission of the Editor, *British Journal of Bone and Joint Surgery,* from Connor and Evans 1982a.)

Short thumbs are also a feature of FOP. The reported incidence of 50%–59% may be an underestimate as this feature is easily overlooked, especially in young children (Fairbank 1950, Schroeder and Zasloff 1980). The thumbs usually have normal mobility, but may stiffen in some patients (Michelson 1904). Clinodactyly, or incurving of the little fingers, occurs in 50% of patients with FOP (Fig. 4.3,

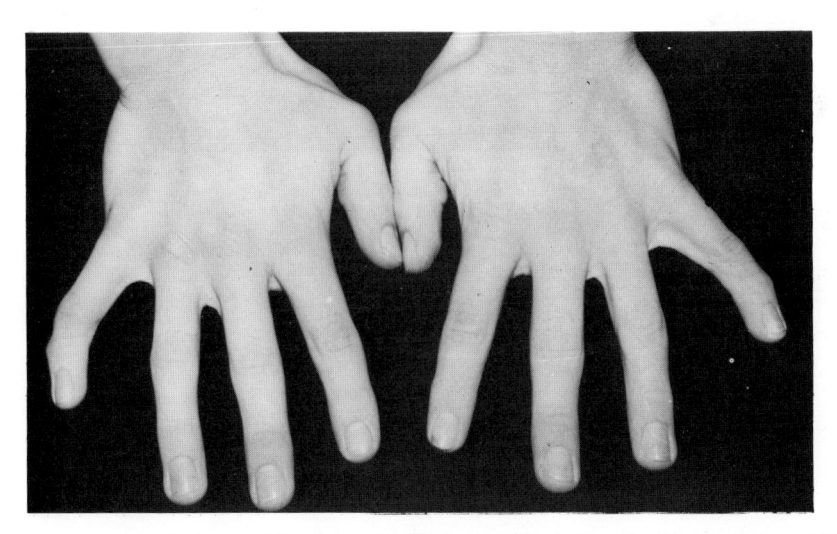

Fig.4.3. Short thumbs and incurving of fifth fingers. (Reproduced with permission of the Editor, *British Journal of Bone and Joint Surgery*, from Connor and Evans 1982a.)

Tünte et al. 1967). Occasionally, shortening or stiffening of other digits may be apparent. All of these digital changes in FOP show striking bilateral symmetry. The changes in the hands lend further support to the diagnosis of FOP but are not specific as similar findings may be seen in the de Lange syndrome.

The pregnancy, birth history and birth weight are unremarkable. Although the digital changes are generally noted at birth, their significance is usually overlooked. Typically, a misdiagnosis of isolated congenital hallux valgus is made; however, in this condition two phalanges are present in each big toe (Kelikian 1965). The child is otherwise asymptomatic until soft tissue ossification occurs.

Ectopic bone formation in FOP usually presents as a series of lumps in the muscles of the neck or back (Fig. 4.4). Ectopic ossification is usually clinically evident by 10 years (Lutwak 1964) and may occasionally be present at birth (Hutchinson 1860, Mair 1932, Connor and Evans 1982a—patient 8). Rarely, the onset of ectopic ossification has been after 20 years of age (Frejka 1929, Friend 1951, Harris 1961). The mean age of onset was 3 years 11 months in the series of Rogers and Geho (1979) and 3 years in the UK series.

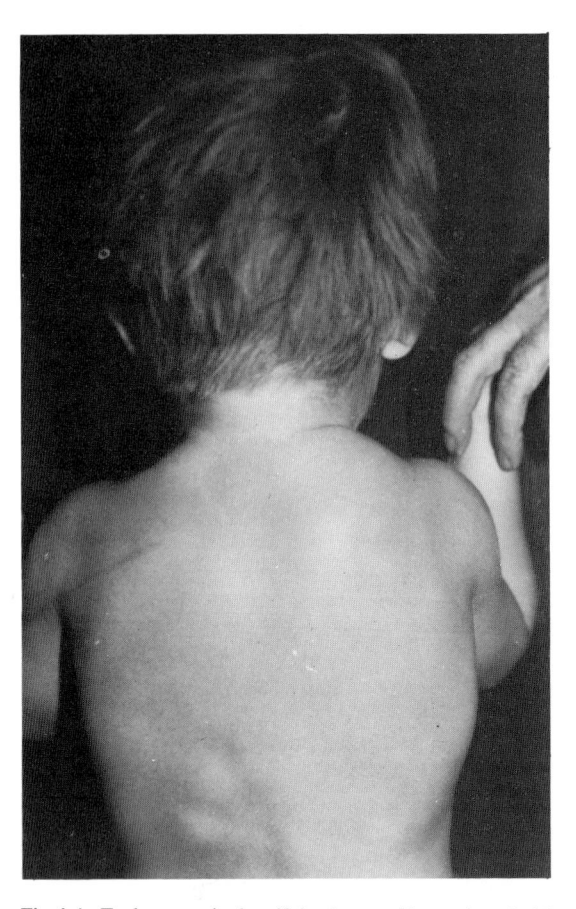

Fig.4.4. Early paraspinal ossifying lumps. (Reproduced with permission of the Editor, *British Journal of Bone and Joint Surgery*, from Connor and Evans 1982a.)

Clinical Features 59

Ossifying lumps appear over several hours, tend to be asymmetric and are variable in both size and shape. They may, or may not, be painful and the overlying skin may be warm and reddened (Smith 1975). Lumps are usually firm in texture and gradually shrink in size over several days or weeks (Garrod 1907). They may be succeeded by other lumps and this often gives the patient the mistaken impression that the lumps are moving about (Mair 1932). Occasionally, fever or malaise accompanies the appearance of new lumps but generally constitutional disturbance is absent (Fairbank 1950).

The lumps themselves cause stiffness, which improves as they subside, but the disease process continues and when ectopic bone forms, irreversible limitation of movement becomes apparent (Smith 1975, Fig. 4.5).

Lumps are usually spontaneous but local trauma is a well-recognized precipitating factor (Mair 1932, McKusick 1972). Such local trauma includes: intramuscular injections (Akin et al. 1975); lump biopsy (Makhani 1970); operations to excise ectopic bone (Rogers and Geho 1979); accidental injury; dental therapy; and careless venepuncture (Connor and Evans 1982a). Local trauma, although an important avoidable precipitating factor, does not invariably result in an exacerbation and it should be emphasized that the majority of episodes of ossification occur without apparent provocation.

Ectopic bone formation in FOP has a predilection for certain sites. The axial musculature bears the brunt of the disease and limb involvement tends to be most marked proximally (Lutwak 1964). Further, proximal muscle involvement tends

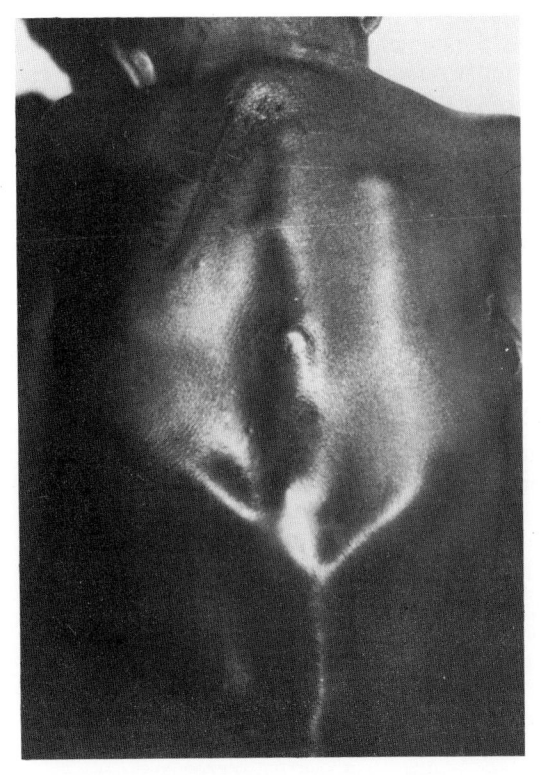

Fig. 4.5. Mature paraspinal ectopic bone.

to precede distal. The muscles of mastication are also a common site of involvement (Connor and Evans 1982c). Involvement of the muscles of the anterior abdominal wall is infrequent (Griffith 1949) and involvement of the muscles of facial expression is rare (McKusick 1972—case 4). Curiously, certain muscles are never involved. These include: the tongue, extraocular muscles, larynx, diaphragm, sphincter muscles and visceral smooth muscle.

Ectopic bone formation also occurs in ligaments, fasciae, aponeuroses, tendon and joint capsules. Although skin ossification has only been recorded once (Rosenstirn 1918), pressure ulceration over a projecting mass of bone is not infrequent (Fairbank 1950). The skin has normal elasticity and skin wounds heal normally without ossifying. Bone formation has never been recorded in the viscera, including the heart.

Stiffness of the cervical spine is a common early finding (Connor and Smith 1982). Later, fixation of major joints results in a progressive reduction in mobility and unusual movements are developed to help accomplish daily requirements (Smith 1975). A few patients present only with progressive stiffness and do not recall acute ossifying lumps. Costovertebral joint involvement results in restricted chest expansion and patients depend upon the function of the uninvolved diaphragm for respiration (Connor et al. 1981).

Deafness is a feature of FOP. This was first noted by Lutwak (1964) and was present in 28% (12 of 42) of the patients of Rogers and Geho (1979) and 24% (8 of 34) of the UK patients. When audiometry has been performed, the deafness has usually been conductive (Lutwak 1964, Letts 1968, Ludman et al. 1968). Onset of deafness is often in adolescence or early adult life. It develops over a period of some weeks and is then non-progressive. This deafness may be secondary to middle ear ossification but in the only patient who had surgical exploration of the middle ear, a mobile ossicular chain and no evidence of stapedius ossification were found (Ludman et al. 1968). Ocular problems do not occur in FOP and mental development is usually normal. Two patients in the series of Connor and Evans (1982a) were mildly mentally retarded: interestingly these two also had the most severe hand and foot malformations with reduction defects of all digits.

Failure of secondary sexual development is considered by some to be a common feature (Rosenstirn 1918, Riley and Christie 1951, Tünte et al. 1967) but this view is not shared by all authors (Fairbank 1950). Sexual development was normal in all males of the UK series and only one female failed to develop normal secondary sexual characteristics. Menstrual irregularities and premature menopause were, however, frequent and the endocrinological basis for this merits further investigation. Longitudinal growth is normal, but true stature may be masked by joint ankylosis. Excessive skin seborrhea has been an occasional feature (Maudsley 1952, Letts 1968, Connor, 1981).

In the UK series, 24% (8 of 34) had diffuse scalp baldness. This was all the more remarkable since the majority of these bald patients were female and had noted hair thinning from middle age. This hair loss could not be explained by medications or poor nutritional status. Eyebrows, eyelashes, axillary and pubic hair were not involved. This has not previously been stressed as a feature of FOP, but is evident in several of the older case descriptions (Burton-Fanning and Vaughan 1901, Frejka 1929, Letts 1968).

Despite this characteristic clinical picture, delay in diagnosis is almost invariable: abnormal, especially monophalangic, big toes in a patient with soft tissue ossification should always suggest FOP.

Radiology

The radiological findings in FOP illustrate the combination of skeletal malformations, ectopic ossification, and skeletal changes secondary to immobilization and therapy.

The skeletal malformations are widespread and in addition to changes in the digits include: short broad femoral necks, shallow acetabulae, mis-shapen cervical vertebrae and short mandibular necks (Letts 1968, Cremin et al. 1982). The changes in the cervical spine were first emphasized by Hall and Sutcliffe (1979) and consist of small bodies, enlarged pedicles and 'massive' spinous processes. Progressive fusion of both the bodies and the apophyseal joints is later superimposed (Figs. 4.6 and 4.7, Connor and Smith 1982).

In the hands, the commonest findings are short first metacarpals and malformed middle phalanges of the fifth fingers with clinodactyly. The changes in the feet are more variable and have been reviewed by several authors (McKusick 1972, Smith 1975, Schroeder and Zasloff 1980, Connor and Evans 1982a). Commonly, only a single phalanx is present in each big toe. In early childhood an accessory epiphysis may be present near the head of each first metatarsal which may later fuse to either the phalanx or the metatarsal (Figs. 4.8 and 4.9). Some patients have two malformed phalanges in each big toe which later fuse (Fig. 4.10), and occasionally the initial radiographs of the feet are completely normal. Synostosis of the phalanges both of the big toe and of the thumb often occurs in later

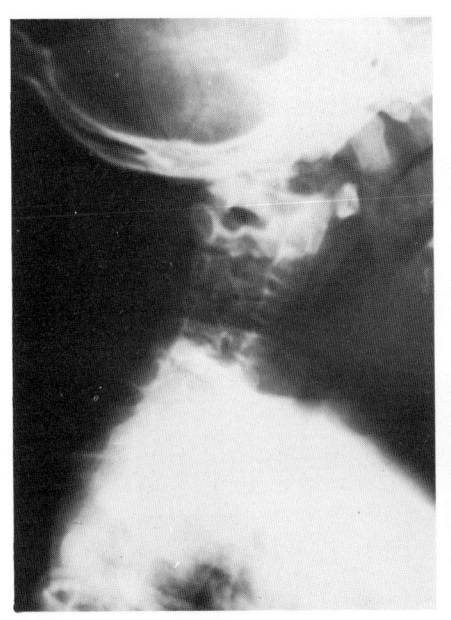

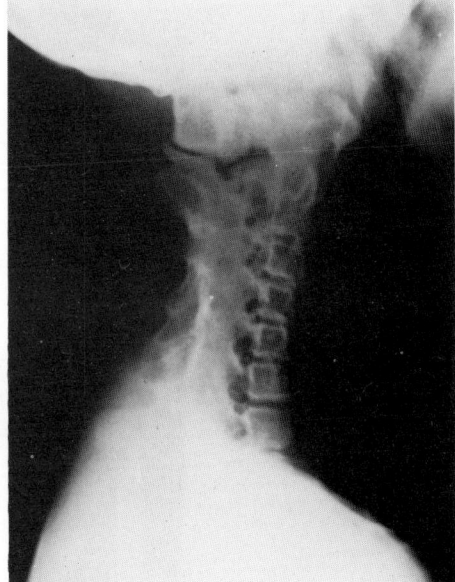

Fig.4.6. (*left*) Malformed cervical vertebrae in a 1-year-old. (Reproduced with permission of the Editor, *British Journal of Radiology*, from Connor and Smith 1982.)

Fig.4.7. (*right*) Extensive cervical fusion at 10 years of age: same patient as Fig. 4.6. (Reproduced with permission of the Editor, from Connor and Smith 1982.)

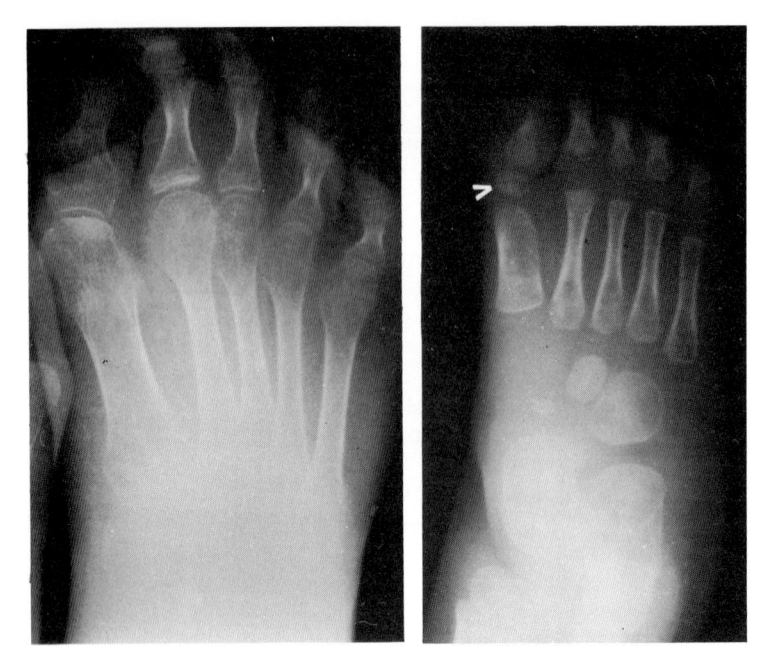

Fig.4.8. (*left*) Monophalangic big toe with valgus deviation. (Reproduced with permission of the Editor, *British Journal of Bone and Joint Surgery*, from Connor and Evans 1982a.)
Fig.4.9. (*right*) Accessory epiphysis (arrowed) in the monophalangic big toe of a 2-year-old.

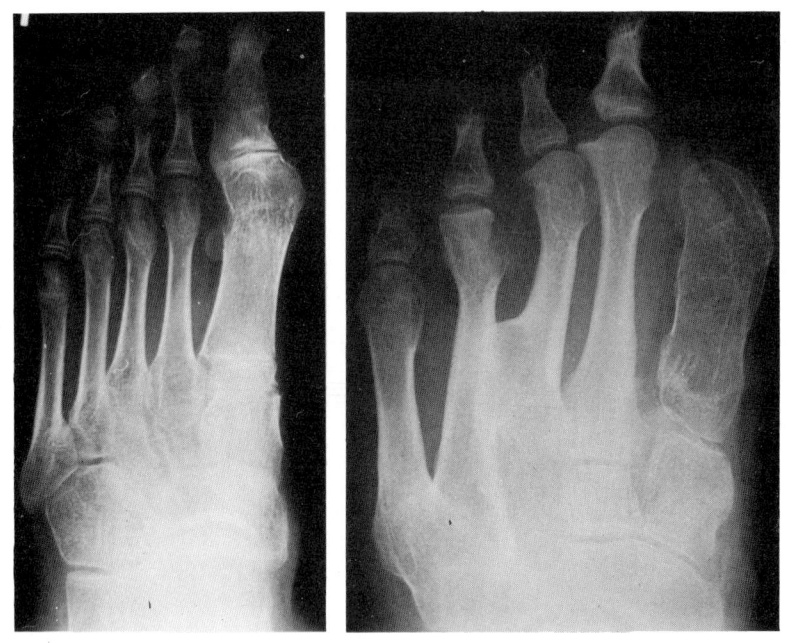

Fig.4.10. (*left*) Fusion of two malformed phalanges of big toe in a 14-year-old.
Fig.4.11. (*right*) Reduction defects of all digits. (Reproduced with permission of the Editor, *British Journal of Bone and Joint Surgery*, from Connor and Evans 1982a.)

childhood. Schroeder and Zasloff (1980) found synostosis of other toes in half of their patients. Occasional patients have severe reduction defects of all digits. In contrast to the soft tissue ossification these skeletal malformations tend to show marked bilateral symmetry.

Ectopic bone is apparent on radiographs 2–8 months after the initial appearance of an ossifying lump (Riley and Christie 1951). This matures and develops normal trabecular architecture (Fig. 4.12). Initial development occurs in the skeletal muscles, but secondary attachment to the skeleton is common (Fig. 4.13). Ectopic bone also develops in ligaments and tendons: this is believed to account for the 'exostoses' which are a common feature of FOP (Cremin et al. 1982). Ectopic bone behaves as normal bone on a bone scan (Holan et al. 1973). Computerized tomography confirms that the initial lesions develop in the intermuscular connective tissue (M. A. Zasloff 1982, personal communication).

Immobilization results in osteoporosis and this is most marked in the region of ankylosed joints (Fig. 4.14). Occasionally, pathological fractures may ensue (Münchmeyer 1869). Corticosteroid therapy may enhance this osteoporosis. Diphosphonate therapy may produce widening of the physis and disorganized metaphyseal bone growth (Wood and Robinson 1976).

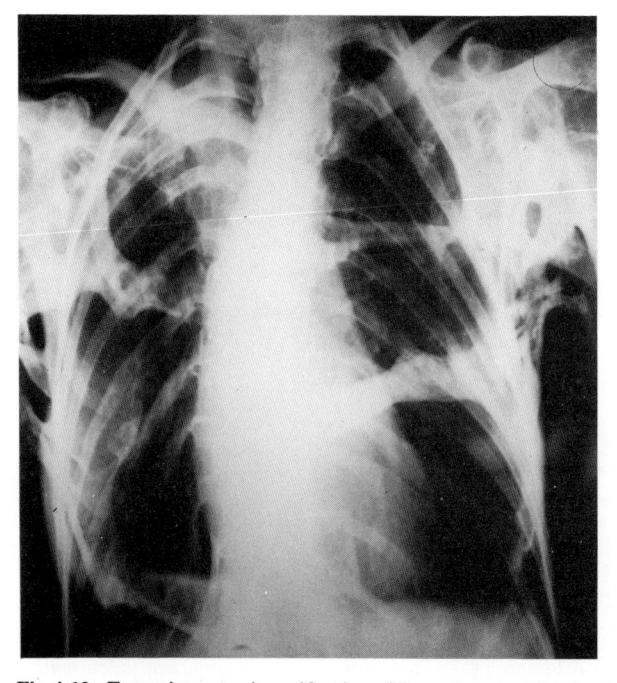

Fig.4.12. Extensive ectopic ossification. (Reproduced with permission of the Editor, *Thorax*, from Connor et al. 1981.)

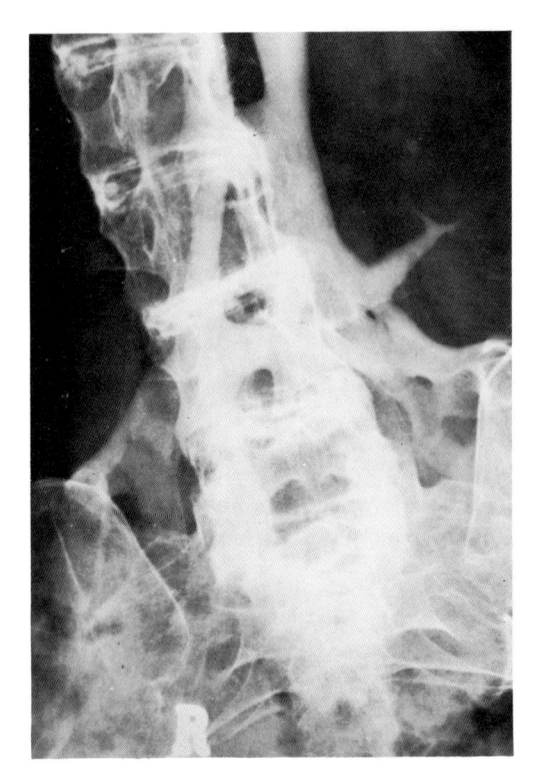

Fig.4.13. Paraspinal ossification of ligaments and muscle connective tissue.

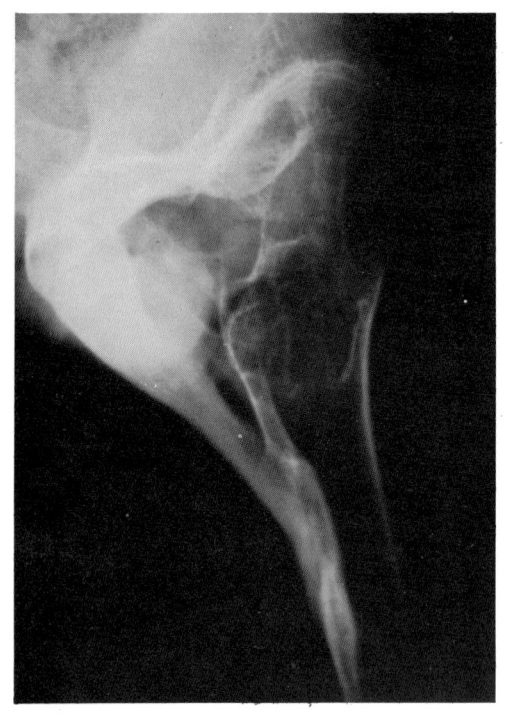

Fig.4.14. Ankylosis of the hip with disuse osteoporosis. (Reproduced with permission of the Editor, *British Journal of Bone and Joint Surgery*, from Connor and Evans 1982a.)

Laboratory Studies

In contrast with the striking clinical and radiological findings, results of routine biochemical tests are normal in FOP.

Serum calcium, phosphate, and alkaline phosphatase levels are normal, provided age-matched controls are used (Smith 1975). Indeed total body calcium metabolism appears to be normal (Austin 1907, Lutwak 1964). Results of the following tests have repeatedly been found to be normal: urinanalysis, full blood count, erythrocyte sedimentation rate, coagulation studies, serum urea and electrolytes, serum magnesium, muscle enzymes, liver function, thyroid function and electrophoresis of plasma proteins. The karyotype, on both lymphocytes and cultured skin fibroblasts, is normal (Tünte et al. 1967, Letts 1968, Connor 1981). In one patient nerve conduction studies were performed and were normal (Letts 1968). Connor (1981) noted no difference in the distribution of histocompatibility antigens between 22 FOP patients and 550 normal controls.

Urinary excretion of hydroxyproline, as a measure of collagen turnover, is usually normal (Smith et al. 1976) although increased values have been occasionally noted (Blumenkrantz and Asboe-Hansen 1978). To date there have been relatively few studies of tissue collagen in FOP. Francis et al. (1973) reported increased extraction of soluble collagen from a skin sample from one FOP patient and thought this might represent reduced collagen cross-linking. This technique can, however, produce misleading results as it is highly dependent upon the exact conditions of extraction. Gay and Miller (1978) used immunological detection to study collagen production in FOP. The new fibrous tissue between the degenerating muscle cells was found to be replaced by ectopic cartilage containing type II collagen. This was followed by cartilage resorption and deposition of calcified bone matrix containing type I collagen. These changes are identical to those which occur during normal enchondral ossification. More recently, a normal collagen pattern of types I and III has been demonstrated using SDS electrophoresis in an ossifying lump in FOP (Burow et al. 1980).

Several patients with FOP have had abnormal electrocardiograms which included bundle branch block and ST segment changes (Campbell 1933, Lutwak 1964, Fletcher and Moss 1965, Connor et al. 1981).

Pulmonary function tests reveal abnormalities even in childhood, and show a restrictive ventilatory defect and reduced lung volumes (Weiss et al. 1971, Bland et al. 1973, Suzuki et al. 1976, Hentzer et al. 1977a, Connor et al. 1981). Despite this chest wall restriction, arterial blood gases have been normal in the few cases where they have been measured (Schönthal 1967, Letts 1968, Buhain et al. 1974, Connor et al. 1981).

Pathology

The pathological features depend upon the stage of the disease. Muscles are histologically normal prior to involvement (McKusick 1972). This was questioned by Smith et al. (1966) who found a myopathic electromyogram and an abnormal muscle biopsy, with variable fiber size and reduced ATPase, before evidence of muscle ossification. However, their patient had generalized muscle weakness and reduced tendon reflexes: findings which are not features of FOP. Thus, it would appear that their patient had a coexistent myopathy, and subsequent electromyograms from uninvolved areas in FOP patients have been normal (Hentzer et al. 1977a).

In the early stages the involved muscles are yellowish-red, soft, swollen and edematous (Riley and Christie 1951). At this stage there is considerable proliferation of connective tissue between the bundles of striated muscle (Fig. 4.15, Weber and Compton 1914, Eaton et al. 1957, Frame et al. 1972, Suzuki et al. 1976). The cellular proliferation is particularly marked about blood vessels and consists mainly of fibroblasts (Fig. 4.16, Eaton et al. 1957).

Wilkins et al. (1935) made the important discovery that these early lumps have extremely high levels of alkaline phosphatase activity. They used a biochemical assay of tissue extracts and noted that the activity was mainly in the fibrous component of the biopsy specimen and was normal in the adjacent normal muscle. These findings have been repeatedly confirmed (Dixon et al. 1954, Lins and Abath 1959, Bona et al. 1967, Mercante and Villani 1967).

Electron microscopy of a lump was performed by Hentzer et al. (1977b). Fibroblasts were the predominant cell type and appeared to be synthetically active as they had extensive endoplasmic reticulum and a large Golgi apparatus. Maxwell et al. (1977) also used electron microscopy on a lump biopsy and noted that the fibroblasts resembled osteoblasts both morphologically and cytochemically. They demonstrated abundant alkaline phosphatase in these cells using histochemical methods. Macrophages were also present in the lump and these were rich in acid phosphatase. Bona et al. (1967) also noted high levels of alkaline phosphatase in the ectopic osteoblasts and commented that the profile of activity of other enzymes was typical of that seen at sites of normal bone formation.

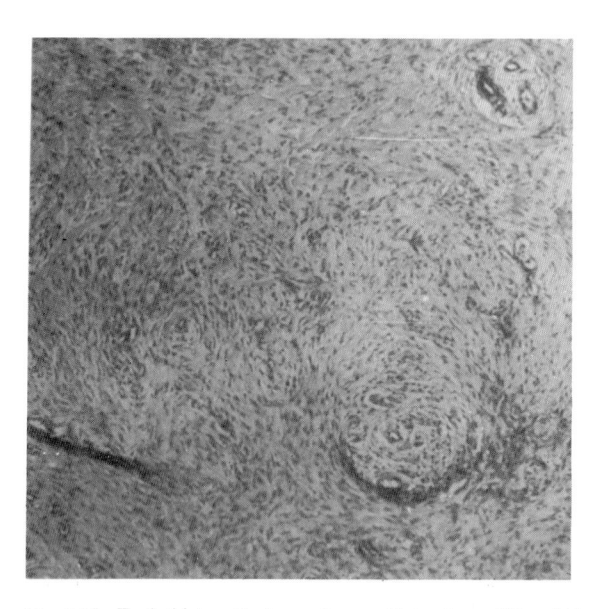

Fig.4.15. Early histopathology of an ossifying lump (H and E, ×75).

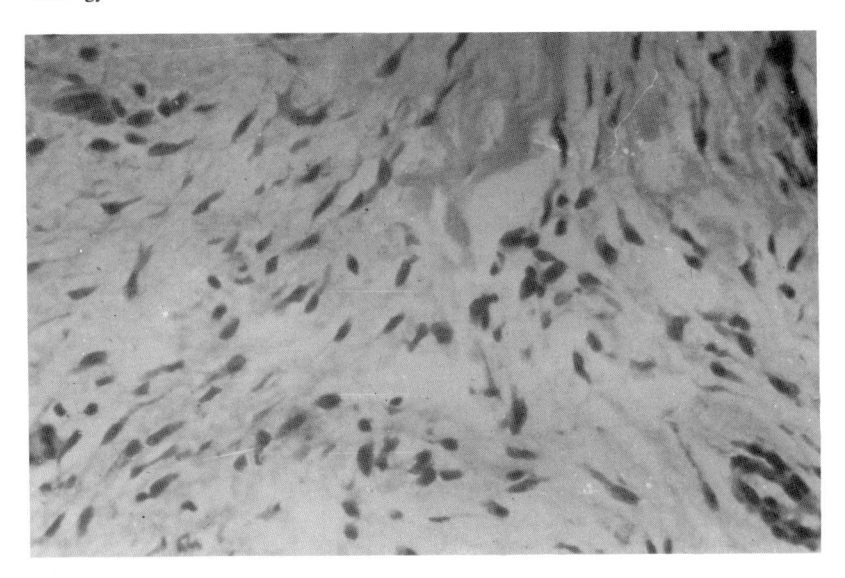

Fig.4.16. Early histopathology of an ossifying lump (H and E, ×250).

The muscle fibers may show signs of degeneration even in the early stages, with loss of striations and flocculation of proteins within the sarcolemma (Eaton et al. 1957). Cartilage is often found in the later lesions but bone may also form by intramembranous ossification (Riley and Christie 1951, Bona et al. 1967). Later in the disease, mature lamellar bone is found which is histologically indistinguishable from normal bone and contains osteoblasts, osteocytes, osteoclasts, Haversian systems and marrow (Fairbank 1950, Maudsley 1952, Suzuki et al. 1976). Bone may lie free in the muscles or fuse with adjacent parts of the skeleton. The ectopic bone does not conform to the outlines of the muscles from which it arises (Webb 1953).

Since pathological changes in FOP primarily affect connective tissue, several authors have studied FOP fibroblasts in vitro. Fibroblasts grown from an ossifying lump have high levels of alkaline phosphatase activity whereas fibroblasts from uninvolved areas have normal levels of activity, provided age-matched controls are used (Herrman et al. 1969, Beratis et al. 1976, Miller et al. 1977, Connor and Evans 1981). Maxwell et al. (1978) noted that cells from an ossifying lesion synthesize in vitro large amounts of a material like prostaglandin E. However, addition of prostaglandin E to non-lesion cells did not result in an increase in alkaline phosphatase activity.

Etiology

FOP is inherited as an autosomal dominant trait with full penetrance but variable expression (Connor and Evans 1982b). The few patients with FOP who have reproduced, have produced affected offspring (Sympson 1886, Burton-Fanning and Vaughan 1901, Rivalta 1902, Gaster 1905, Painter and Clarke 1909, Drago 1919, Decastello 1954, Gorynski and Litynska 1958, Harris 1961, Logacev 1964, McKusick 1972). Gaster (1905) briefly described a family in which members of three generations were affected. Further, support for the genetic etiology is provided by the two reported sets of concordant monozygotic twins (Vastine et al. 1948, Eaton et al. 1957).

As FOP patients rarely reproduce, the majority of patients in practise will have normal parents and represent fresh dominant mutations (Tünte et al. 1967). The risk to a normal couple of conceiving a child with FOP thus depends upon the mutation rate, and this risk is further increased with increasing age of the father. This paternal age effect for new FOP mutations has been shown in Germany (Tünte et al. 1967), the USA (Rogers and Chase 1979) and the UK (Connor and Evans 1982b). A paternal age effect has also been shown for new mutations in at least 12 other autosomal dominant disorders (Jones et al. 1975).

The mutation rate for FOP was estimated in Merseyside, UK, as 1.8×10^{-6} mutations per gene per generation (Connor and Evans 1982b). If this is applicable to the whole of the UK there should be 1 or 2 new cases per year in the UK. Similarly there should be 4 or 5 new cases per year in the USA. The geographical distribution of new cases in the UK revealed clustering, but this conformed to the population distribution as a whole.

In pigs FOP is also inherited as an autosomal dominant trait, with 35 of 115 offspring of a male proband affected (Seibold and Davis 1967).

Although FOP is inherited as a mendelian autosomal dominant trait, the actual mechanism by which the mutant gene produces it effects, or indeed the function of the normal gene, is unknown. An abnormality of calcium or phosphate metabolism has been proposed on several occasions (Mair 1932, Dixon et al. 1954). There is no evidence to support this in FOP, and diseases with such disturbances result in metastatic calcification not ossification (Chap. 1). Collagen structure may be abnormal in FOP and thus favor ossification at abnormal sites (Lutwak 1964, McKusick 1972, Blumenkrantz and Asboe-Hansen 1978). This might also account for the association with skeletal malformations. However, recent studies on collagen structure provide no support for this hypothesis (Burow et al. 1980).

Herrman et al. (1969) proposed that the digital malformations might result from ectopic ossification in utero. This seems unlikely, as ectopic ossification is rarely evident in infancy and is usually asymmetric, whereas the skeletal malformations are congenital and symmetric. Schroeder and Zasloff (1980) suggested that the defective gene might produce its effects by failure to act at the critical phase for digital formation (days 43 to 44 of intra-uterine life), but this ignores the more widespread skeletal malformations and gives no clue as to the mechanism of the ectopic ossification.

Virchow (1894) believed that there was a disturbance of embryonic development with resultant intramuscular periosteal rests which then exerted an osteogenic influence on the adjacent normal muscle fibroblasts. Other authors have suggested an abnormal persistence of mesenchymal cells which themselves have the capability of becoming osteoblasts (Paget 1895, Rolleston 1901, Bona et al. 1967). However, it is now suspected that normal individuals have mesenchymal cells, the inducible osteogenic precursor cells, which under certain conditions can differentiate into osteoblasts. These cells are present in several types of connective tissue but are most frequent in the connective tissue of skeletal muscles (see p. 109). The primary fault in FOP probably represents a genetic defect in the normal regulatory mechanisms of these cells. However, the nature of these regulatory mechanisms is as yet unknown (Chaps. 7 and 8).

Natural History

Erratic progression of disability is usual in FOP. Rogers and Geho (1979) could only conclude that the oldest patients tended to be most disabled. All patients in the UK series had long periods of apparent disease inactivity but certain generalizations were possible: all patients had limitation of spine and both shoulders by 10 years; one or both hips were involved by 20 years of age; and most were chair-bound or bed-bound by 30 years of age (Connor and Evans 1982a). Progression of disability was not influenced by sex; place of birth or residence; age at, or site of, onset; type or extent of skeletal malformations; or the presence of medical therapy. Ectopic ossification, though generally less active in adults, does not stop completely and continues into old age (Smith 1975, Connor and Evans 1982a). Occasionally, temporary improvement occurs as a result of fracture in an area of ectopic bone and the formation of a false joint, but few, if any, would agree with Mair's statement (1932) that disease regression is a frequent occurrence. Fairbank (1950) observed that there had been no recorded case of recovery from FOP and this conclusion is still valid.

Although lifespan is reduced in FOP, most patients will reach adult life. In the UK series the age range was 4 to 70 years with a mean of 28 years and the average age at death in 33 reported cases was 34.7 years (Connor 1981). Thus the view of some authors (Mair 1932, Griffith 1949, Sastri and Yadav 1977) that the majority will die under 15 years of age appears unduly pessimistic (the patient who was reported by Griffith at 3 years of age is currently chair-bound but 33 years old). Several FOP patients have reached old age despite their physical handicaps (Opie 1917, McKusick 1972—patient 5). The average lifespan for a FOP patient is probably about 35 years.

Pneumonia is the usual terminal illness and this is favored by the chest wall restriction. Some authors suggest that chronic respiratory failure may occur, but this is not supported by the lack of progression in chest wall restriction during adult life and the limited observations to date on arterial blood gases (Connor et al. 1981).

Occasional patients die from starvation secondary to jaw fixation, from accidental injury or by suicide (Tutunjian and Kegerreis 1937). One patient in the UK series who died of pneumonia had partial atlanto-axial subluxation at autopsy. Pack and Braund (1942) reported malignant transformation to a myxoliposarcoma in a 7-year-old boy with FOP. These authors did not, however, provide long-term follow-up and the interpretation of the histopathology of the early FOP lesions is often confused with sarcoma or congenital fibromatosis (Chap. 1).

Management

The diagnosis of FOP should be made on the basis of the clinical and radiological findings. Lump biopsy is unnecessary and should be avoided as it often exacerbates local bone production.

Treatment of FOP is fraught with difficulties. The pathogenesis of the disease is not known and thus therapy has necessarily been largely empirical. The disease course is naturally erratic and unpredictable, and this hampers assessment of potential therapies (Illingworth 1971). Controlled trials would be desirable, but as the disease is rare, these would be difficult to organize and have not as yet been undertaken. Numerous remedies have been tried at various times (Table 4.1), but none of these has been of proven value (Connor and Evans 1982a).

Table 4.1. Unsuccessful therapies for fibrodysplasia ossificans progressiva.

Physical agents	Bathing, bleeding, ice, hot air, local blisters, ultrasound
Special diets	Low calcium, low vitamin D, ketogenic
Vitamins	B, E
Acids	Hydrochloric, nitric, lactic, phosphoric
Hormones	Thyroid extract, parathyroid extract, corticosteroids, androgens, estrogens, propylthiouracil, anabolic steroids
Surgery	Excision of ectopic bone, thymectomy, parathyroidectomy
Radiation	Radiotherapy, local radium implants, mesothorium
Medications	Disodium etidronate, EDTA, D-penicillamine, colchicum, salicylates, antimitotics, fibrinolysins, sodium citrate, disodium hydrogen phosphate, thiosamine
Others	Mercury, iodides, arsenic, beryllium, sarsparilla

Three therapies merit further comment: corticosteroids, excision of ectopic bone and diphosphonates. Corticosteroids have now been used for more than 20 years in the treatment of FOP patients and have not produced any objective benefit (Riley and Christie 1951, Dixon et al. 1954, Illingworth 1971). Many FOP patients have had ectopic bone excised. Recurrence within 4 months has been the usual result (Mair 1932, Riley and Christie 1951, Maudsley 1952, Dixon et al. 1954, Holmsen et al. 1979), and only occasionally has bone failed to recur at the operation site (Russell et al. 1972). Rogers and Geho (1979) reported on 55 operations or biopsy procedures on 37 FOP patients: 34 operations resulted in increased disability and only 6 produced benefit (and of these, 3 were for correction of hallux valgus). Surgery is, however, useful in allowing refixation of a joint in an improved functional position. Curiously, ossification is not a problem after abdominal surgery for intercurrent illness.

Recently, diphosphonates, notably disodium etidronate (EHDP), have been evaluated in FOP. Diphosphonates inhibit the formation and dissolution of hydroxyapatite, both in vitro and in vivo (Francis et al. 1969). Unfortunately, the initial encouraging reports (Bassett et al. 1969, Weiss et al. 1971, Geho and Whiteside 1973) have not been followed by evidence for long-term benefit. Whilst continued, this therapy does inhibit calcification, but does not halt production of the ectopic bone matrix which itself is disabling (Russell et al. 1972—case 1). In addition, it also inhibits mineralization of the normal bone and may result in undesirable skeletal side-effects (Wood and Robinson 1976). Thus at the present time, no form of medical therapy is know to be of benefit and surgical removal of ectopic bone may do more harm than good.

Patients should be informed of the avoidable factors which can precipitate ossification, including: local muscle trauma, careless venepuncture, intramuscular injections, lump biopsy and operations to excise ectopic bone. Dental therapy should be approached with caution and anesthetists need to be warned of the possibility of atlanto-axial subluxation and that endotracheal intubation may be technically difficult because of jaw fixation. There is no evidence that physical exercise or physiotherapy have an adverse or favorable influence on the progression of this disease.

As death is usually due to pneumonia, attention should be directed towards prevention and therapy of intercurrent chest infections. Such measures might include: chest physiotherapy; prompt antibiotic therapy of early infection; and prophylaxis with pneumoccal and influenzal vaccines. Obviously, factors which interfere with diaphragmatic respiration, such as upper abdominal surgery, should be avoided if possible. Similarly, fixation of the spine with a high thoracic scoliosis should be avoided or corrected if possible, since this will further compromise pulmonary function.

General measures designed to help patients cope with physical disability, such as aids for everyday tasks, adapting the environment and the provision of appropriate wheelchairs, will be required. Complete management should include genetic counseling for patients and their families.

References

Akin RK, Keller AJ, Walters PJ (1975) Myositis ossificans progressiva: A diagnostic problem. J Oral Surg 33: 611–615
Austin AE (1907) Calcium metabolism in a case of myositis ossificans. J Med Res (Boston) 16: 451–458
Bassett CAL, Donath A, Macagno F, Preisig R, Fleisch H, Francis MD (1969) Diphosphonates in the treatment of myositis ossificans (letter). Lancet II: 845
Bauer KH, Bode W (1940) Erbpathologie der Stützgewebe beim Menschen. Julius Springer, Berlin (Handbuch der Erbbiologie des Menschen, vol 3, p 105)
Beratis NG, Kaffe S, Aron AM, Hirschhorn K (1976) Alkaline phosphatase activity in cultured skin fibroblasts from fibrodysplasia ossificans progressiva. J Med Genet 13: 307–309
Bland JH, Kirschbaum B, O'Connor GT, Whorton E (1973) Myositis ossificans progressiva. Effect of intravenously given parathyroid extract on urinary excretion of connective tissue components. Arch Intern Med 132: 209–212
Blumenkrantz N, Asboe-Hansen G (1978) Fibrodysplasia ossificans progressiva. Biochemical changes in blood, serum, urine, skin, bone and ectopic ossification. Scand J Rheumatol 7: 85–89
Bona C, Stanescu V, Dumitrescu MS, Ionescu V (1967) Histochemical and cytoenzymological studies in myositis ossificans. Acta Histochem 27: 207–224
Buhain WJ, Rammohan G, Berger HW (1974) Pulmonary function in myositis ossificans progressiva. Am Rev Respir Dis 110: 333–337
Burow HM, Jonak R, Sauer O, Diehm T (1980) Myositis ossificans progressiva (MOP). Eine morphologische und biochemische Studie. Klin Paediatr 192: 467–473
Burton-Fanning FW, Vaughan AL (1901) A case of myositis ossificans. Lancet II: 849–850
Campbell RK (1933) Myositis ossificans progressiva. Radiol Rev 55: 153–156
Connor JM (1981) A national investigation into the clinical, genetic and pathogenetic aspects of fibrodysplasia ossificans progressiva. MD thesis, University of Liverpool
Connor JM, Evans DAP (1981) Quantitative and qualitative studies on fibroblast alkaline phosphatase in fibrodysplasia ossificans progressiva. Clin Chim Acta 117: 355–360

Connor JM, Evans DAP (1982a) Fibrodysplasia ossificans progressiva. The clinical features and natural history of 34 patients. J Bone Joint Surg [Br] 64: 76–83

Connor JM, Evans DAP (1982b) Genetic aspects of fibrodysplasia ossificans progessiva. J Med Genet 19: 35–39

Connor JM, Evans DAP (1982c) Extra-articular ankylosis in fibrodysplasia ossificans progressiva. Br J Oral Surg 20: 117–121

Connor JM, Smith R (1982) The cervical spine in fibrodysplasia ossificans progressiva. Br J Radiol 55: 492–496

Connor JM, Evans CC, Evans DAP (1981) Cardiopulmonary function in fibrodysplasia ossificans progressiva. Thorax 36: 419–423

Cremin B, Connor JM, Beighton P (1982) The radiological spectrum of fibrodysplasia ossificans progressiva. Clin Radiol 33: 499–508

Decastello A (1954) Osteomyelosklerose bei Vater und Tochter. Wien Klin Wochnschr 66: 655–658

Dixon TF, Mulligan L, Nassim R, Stevenson FH (1954) Myositis ossificans progressiva. Report of a case in which ACTH and cortisone failed to prevent reossification after excision of ectopic bone. J Bone Joint Surg [Br] 36: 445–449

Drago A (1919) Contributo all studio della miosite ossificante progressive multipla (Malatti di Münchmeyer). Pediatria Napoli 27: 715–753

Eaton WL, Conkling WS, Daeschner CW (1957) Early myositis ossificans progressiva occurring in homozygotic twins. A clinical and pathologic study. J Pediatr 50: 591–598

Ebrahim GJ, Grech P, Slavin G (1966) Myositis ossificans progressiva in an African child. Br J Radiol 39: 952–953

Fairbank HAT (1950) Myositis ossificans progressiva. J Bone Joint Surg [Br] 32: 108–116

Fleissner HK (1975) Zur myositis ossificans progressiva. Beitr Orthop Traumatol 22: 48–51

Fletcher E, Moss MS (1965) Myositis ossificans progressiva. Ann Rheum Dis 24: 267–272

Frame B, Azad N, Reynolds WA, Saeed SM (1972) Polyostotic fibrous dysplasia and myositis ossificans progressiva. A report of coexistence. Am J Dis Child 124: 120–122

Francis MD, Russell RGG, Fleisch H (1969) Diphosphonates inhibit formation of calcium phosphate crystals in vitro and pathological calcification in vivo. Science 165: 1264–1266

Francis MJO, Smith R, MacMillan DC (1973) Polymeric collagen of skin in normal subjects and in patients with inherited connective tissue disorders. Clin Sci 44: 429–438

Frejka B (1929) Heterotopic ossification and myositis ossificans progressiva. J Bone Joint Surg 27: 157–166

Freke J (1736) A case of an extraordinary exostosis on the back of a boy. Philos Trans R Soc Lond 1735–1743; 41: 413

Friend J (1951) Myositis ossificans progressiva. Arch Middlesex Hosp 1: 208–212

Garrod AE (1907) The initial stages of myositis ossificans progressiva. St Bartholomew's Hosp Rep 43: 43–49

Gaster A (1905) Discussion in meeting of West London Medico-Chirurgical Society, 7 October 1904. West Lond Med J 10: 37

Gay S, Miller EJ (1978) Collagen in the physiology and pathology of connective tissue. Gustav Fischer Verlag, Stuttgart New York

Geho WB, Whiteside JA (1973) Experience with disodium etidronate in diseases of ectopic calcification. In: Frame B, Parfitt AM, Duncan H (eds) International symposium on clinical aspects of metabolic bone disease. American Elsevier, New York, pp 506–511 (International Congress Series, no. 270)

Gerber R (1875) Ueber Myositis ossificans progressiva. Dissert Wuerzburg

Gorynski T, Litynska J (1958) Postpujace skostnenie pozaszkieletowa (MOP) (Münchmeyer's disease) J Chir Narzad Ruchu 23: 343–351

Goto S (1913) Pathologisch-anatomisch und klinische Studien über die sogen. Myositis ossificans progressiva multiplex (Hyperplasia fascialis ossificans progressiva). Arch Klin Chir 100: 732–788

Grewal KS, Das N (1953) Myositis ossificans progressiva. J Bone Joint Surg [Br] 35: 244–246

Greig DM (1931) Clinical observations on the surgical pathology of bone. Oliver and Boyd, Edinburgh

Griffith G (1949) Progressive myositis ossificans: Report of a case. Arch Dis Child 24: 71–74

Hall CM, Sutcliffe J (1979) Fibrodysplasia ossificans progressiva. Ann Radiol 22: 119–123

Harris NH (1961) Myositis ossificans progressiva. Proc R Soc Med 54: 70–71

Helferich H (1879) Ein Fall von sogenannter Myositis ossificans progressiva. Aerztliches Intelligenz-Blatt 45: 485–489

Hentzer B, Jacobsen HH, Asboe-Hansen G (1977a) Fibrodysplasia ossificans progressiva. Scand J Rheum 6: 161–171

Hentzer B, Kobayasi T, Asboe-Hansen G (1977b) Ultrastructure of dermal connective tissue in

References

fibrodysplasia ossificans progressiva. Acta Derm Venereol (Stockh) 57: 477–485
Herrman J, Schuster M, Walker FA, White EF, Opitz JM, Zurheim GM (1969) Fibrodysplasia ossificans progressiva and the XXXXY syndrome in the same sibship. Birth Defects 5: 43–49
Holan J, Galanda V, Buchanec J (1973) Isotopenuntersuchungen bei der fibrodysplasia ossificans progressiva im Kindersalter mittels Radiostrontium. Radiol Diagn (Berl) 14: 719–726
Holmsen H, Ljunghall S, Hierton T (1979) Myositis ossificans progressiva. Clinical and metabolical observation in a case treated with a diphosphonate (EHDP) and surgical removal of ectopic bone. Acta Orthop Scand 50: 33–38
Hutchinson J (1860) Case of multiple exostoses with ossification of fascia in various parts and icthyosis. Med Times and Gazette 1: 317
Illingworth RS (1971) Myositis ossificans progressiva (Münchmeyer's disease). Brief review with report of two cases treated with corticosteroids and observed for 16 years. Arch Dis Child 46: 264–268
Jones KL, Smith DW, Harvey MAS, Hall BD, Quan L (1975) Older paternal age and fresh gene mutation: Data on additional disorders. J Pediatr 86: 85–88
Kelikian H (1965) Hallux valgus and allied deformities of the forefoot. WB Saunders and Co, Philadelphia
Letts RM (1968) Myositis ossificans progressiva. A report of two cases with chromosome studies. Can Med Assoc J 99: 856–862
Lins FM, Abath GM (1959) Doenca ossificante progressiva. Pediatr Pratica 30: 131–144
Logacev KD (1964) Progressive ossification of muscles. Klin Med 42: 106–110
Ludman H, Hamilton EBD, Eade AWT (1968) Deafness in myositis ossificans progressiva. J Laryngol Otol 82: 57–63
Lutwak L (1964) Myositis ossificans progressiva. Mineral, metabolic and radioactive calcium studies of the effects of hormones. Am J Med 37: 269–293
MacKinnon AP (1924) Progressive myositis ossificans: Report of a case and a review of the literature. J Bone Joint Surg 6: 336–343
McKusick VA (1972) Heritable disorders of connective tissue, 4th edn. CV Mosby Co, St Louis, pp 687–702
Mair WF (1932) Myositis ossificans progressiva. Edinb Med J 39: 13–36, 69–92
Makhani JS (1970) Münchmeyer's disease or fibrodysplasia ossificans progressiva. Indian J Pediatr 37: 535–539
Mather JH (1931) Progressive myositis ossificans. Br J Radiol 4: 207–210
Maudsley RH (1952) A case of myositis ossificans progressiva. Br Med J i: 954–956
Maxwell WA, Spicer SS, Miller RL, Halushka PV, Westphal MC, Setser ME (1977) Histochemical and ultrastructural studies in fibrodysplasia ossificans progressiva (myositis ossificans progressiva). Am J Pathol 87: 483–492
Maxwell WA, Halushka PV, Miller RL, Spicer SS, Westphal MC, Penny LD (1978) Elevated prostaglandin production in cultured cells from a patient with fibrodysplasia ossificans progressiva. Prostaglandins 15: 123–129
Mercante G, Villani M (1967) Studio istologico ed istochimico delle fasi iniziali della miosite ossificante. Riv Anat Patol Oncol 30: 287–313
Michelson J (1904) Ein Fall von Myositis ossificans progressiva. Z Orthop Chir 12: 424–443
Miller RL, Maxwell WA, Spicer SS, Halushka PV, Varner HH, Westphal MC (1977) Studies on alkaline phosphatase activity in cultured cells from a patient with fibrodysplasia ossificans progressiva. Lab Invest 37: 254–259
Moodie RL (1927) Studies in paleopathology. XX. Vertebral lesions in the sabre-tooth, Pleistocene of California, resembling so-called myositis ossificans progressiva, compared with certain ossifications in dinosaurs. Ann Med History 9: 91–102
Münchmeyer E (1869) Ueber Myositis ossificans progressiva. Zeitschrift für rationelle Medizin 34: 9–41
OPCS monitor (1979) Mid-1978 population estimates for health areas (reference PP1 79/6). Office of Population, Censuses and Surveys, London
Opie EL (1917) Progressive muscular ossification (progressive ossifying myositis)—a progressive anomaly of osteogenesis. J Med Res 36: 267–275
Pack GT, Braund RR (1942) The development of sarcoma in myositis ossificans. Report of three cases. JAMA 119: 776–779
Paget S (1895) A case of Myositis ossificans. Lancet I: 339–341
Painter CF, Clark JD (1909) Myositis ossificans. Am J Orthop Surg 6: 626–651
Patin G (1692) Lettres choises de feu M. Guy Patin, vol 1. Letter of 27 August 1648 written to AF. P du Laurens, Cologne, p 28

Riley HD Jr, Christie A (1951) Myositis ossificans progressiva. Pediatrics 8: 753–767
Rivalta F (1902) Sulla un caso di miosite ossificante diffusa progressiva. Policlinico (Rome) 9: 147–161
Rogers JG, Chase GA (1979) Paternal age effect in fibrodysplasia ossificans progressiva. J Med Genet 16: 147–148
Rogers JG, Geho WB (1979) Fibrodysplasia ossificans progressiva. A survey of forty-two cases. J Bone Joint Surg [Am] 61: 909–914
Rolleston HD (1901) Progressive myositis ossificans, with references to other developmental diseases of the mesoblast. Clin J 17: 209–214
Rosenstirn J (1918) A contribution to the study of myositis ossificans progressiva. Ann Surg 68: 485–520, 591–637
Russell RGG, Smith R, Bishop MC, Price DA, Squire CM (1972) Treatment of myositis ossificans progressiva with a diphosphonate. Lancet I: 10–11
Ryan KJ (1945) Myositis ossificans progressiva. A review of the literature with report of a case. J Pediatr 27: 348–352
Sastri VRK, Yadav SS (1977) Myositis ossificans progressiva. Int Surg 62: 45–47
Schönthal H (1967) Atemmechanische Probleme bei der Myositis ossificans progressiva. Beitr Kun Erforsch Tuberk 135: 322–324
Schroeder HW, Zasloff M (1980) The hand and foot malformations in fibrodysplasia ossificans progressiva. Johns Hopkins Med J 147: 73–78
Seibold HR, Davis CL (1967) Generalized myositis ossificans (familial) in pigs. Pathol Vet 4: 79–88
Smith DM, Zeman W, Johnston CC Jr, Deiss WP Jr (1966) Myositis ossificans progressiva. Case report with metabolic and histochemical studies. Metabolism 15: 521–528
Smith R (1975) Myositis ossificans progressiva: a review of current problems. Semin Arthritis Rheum 4: 369–380
Smith R, Russell RGG, Woods CG (1976) Myositis ossificans progressiva. Clinical features of eight patients and their response to therapy. J Bone Joint Surg [Br] 58: 48–57
Stewart AM, MacGregor AR (1951) Myositis fibrosa generalista. Arch Dis Child 26: 215–223
Suzuki T, Ishikawa S, Akanuma N, Tsunoda H (1976) Myositis ossificans progressiva with parathyroid hyperplasia and polycystic ovary. Acta Pathol Jpn 26: 251–262
Sympson T (1886) Case of myositis ossificans. Br Med J ii: 1026–1027
Tünte W, Becker PE, von Knorre G (1967) Zur Genetik der Myositis ossificans progressiva. Humangenetik 4: 320–351
Tutunjian KH, Kegerreis R (1937) Myositis ossificans progressiva with report of a case. J. Bone Joint Surg 19: 503–510
Vastine JH, Vastine MF, Arango O (1948) Myositis ossificans progressiva in homozygotic twins. AJR 59: 204–212
Virchow R (1894) Über myositis progressiva ossificans. Berl Klin Wochenschr 32: 727–729
von Dusch (1868) Cited by Vastine et al. (1948) Myositis ossificans progressiva in homozygotic twins. AJR 59: 204–212
Webb R (1953) Fibrositis ossificans progressiva. Aust NZ J Surg 23: 141–144
Weber FP, Compton A (1914) The early development of myositis ossificans progressiva multiplex, illustrated by an apparently congenital or almost congenital case. Br J Child Dis 11: 497–508
Weiss IW, Fisher L, Phang JM (1971) Diphosphonate therapy in a patient with myositis ossificans progressiva. Ann Intern Med 74: 933–936
Wilkins WE, Regen EM, Carpenter GK (1935) Phosphatase studies on biopsy tissue in progressive myositis ossificans. Am J Dis Child 49: 1219–1221
Wood BJ, Robinson GC (1976) Drug induced bone changes in myositis ossificans progressiva. Pediatr Radiol 5: 40–43

5 Ossification in Neurological Conditions

Although best known as a complication of traumatic paraplegia, soft tissue ossification may occur in the aftermath of a variety of neurological conditions. Despite this diversity, similar pathogenic mechanisms seem to be involved in each case and thus there is an advantage in considering all of these conditions under the same headings.

History and Nomenclature

Riedel in 1883 described the first case of ectopic ossification in a paraplegic patient. Occasional similar cases were reported but interest in this condition was really awakened by studies on the large numbers of patients with traumatic paraplegia following injuries sustained during World War I. Déjérine and colleagues (1918, 1919), in a series of classic papers, described the clinical, radiological and pathological features and called the condition 'para-ostéo-arthropathie'. Drehmann in 1927 published the first description of soft tissue ossification after poliomyelitis and subsequently it was realized that ectopic ossification may complicate a wide variety of neurological conditions. Several names have been proposed for this complication: myositis ossificans neurotica (Meyer 1927, Miller and O'Neill 1949); neurogenic ossifying fibromyositis (Soule 1945); neurogenic osteomas (Benassy 1966); heterotopic ossification in paraplegia (Damanski 1961); and para-articular ossification in spinal cord injury (Freehafer et al. 1966).

Prevalence

The prevalence depends upon the type of neurological lesion, as detailed in Tables 5.1 and 5.2. The reported prevalence in paraplegic patients varied from 4% to 60.5% with most series identifying ectopic bone in 20%–30% of patients. To some extent this wide range reflects differing criteria for diagnosis and differences in protocol for seeking this complication. Stover et al. (1975) conducted a prospective study of 250 cord-injured patients. Serial x-ray films were performed

Table 5.1. Ectopic ossification after paraplegia or quadriplegia.

Series	No. of patients	Prevalence of ossification (%)
Déjérine and Ceillier (1918)	78	49
Soule (1945)	62	37
Heilbrun and Kuhn (1947)	99	44
Abramson (1948)	38	61
Miller and O'Neill (1949)	289	4
Liberson (1953)	30	53
Hardy and Dickson (1963)	603	17
Wright et al. (1965)	38	5
Silver (1969)	124	14
Wharton and Morgan (1970)	447	20
Stover et al. (1975)	250	30
Hassard (1975)	131	47
Scher (1976)	317	20
Hernandez et al. (1978)	704	20
Prakash et al. (1978)	122	33
Blane and Perkash (1981)	376	21

Table 5.2. Ectopic ossification in other neurological conditions.

Series	Diagnosis	No. of patients	Prevalence of ossification (%)
Lorber (1953)	TB meningitis	10	50
Stoikovic et al. (1955)	Poliomyelitis	1980	0.3
Stehman (1959)	Multiple sclerosis	25	24
Hardy and Dixon (1963)	Hemiplegia	500	1
Wharton and Morgan (1970)	Hemiplegia	1911	0.5
Hoffer et al. (1971)	Prolonged coma	122	5
Mendelson et al. (1975)	Prolonged coma	160	22
	Hemiplegia	500	1
Mielants et al. (1975)	Prolonged coma	26	27
Garland et al. (1980)	Prolonged coma	496	11

of the hips, knees, shoulders and elbows. In this carefully conducted study, 76 patients (30%) developed ectopic ossification. The frequency appears to be no different for spastic as compared with flaccid paraplegia. In the series shown in Table 5.1 all patients were adults with traumatic damage to the spinal cord. The cause of the cord damage seems to be less important than the extent of paralysis. Thus, Stehman (1959) found ectopic bone in 6 of 25 patients with quadriplegia secondary to multiple sclerosis. Likewise, Scher (1976) found fewer cases amongst his patients with incomplete cord damage secondary to knife wounds than amongst those patients with complete cord transection. Paraplegia in childhood is relatively uncommon and is more often non-traumatic than in adults. Lorber (1953) reported 10 children with paraplegia secondary to tuberculous meningitis, of whom 5 developed ectopic ossification.

Soft tissue ossification may complicate hemiplegia but is probably much less frequent than after paraplegia, with only 13 cases described up to 1970 (Radt 1970). Mendelson et al. (1975) found ectopic bone in 6 of 500 cases of acute non-traumatic hemiplegia; however, all 6 had been both comatose for a prolonged period and subjected to craniotomy.

Functional paralysis due to prolonged coma of any cause may result in ectopic ossification. Mielants et al. (1975) found ectopic bone in 7 of 26 patients who had long-term coma secondary to head injury. In 5 of these 7 patients, ossification was observed in limbs which were not paralytic and in which integrity of efferent nerve tracts could be demonstrated. Similarly, Mendelson et al. (1975) found ectopic ossification in 35 (22%) of 160 of their patients who had prolonged coma after head trauma, and in a similar group of 496 patients Garland et al. (1980) found 57 (11%) affected. The duration rather than the cause of the coma appears to be the important factor and cases of ectopic bone have been described after coma secondary to encephalitis (Storey and Tegner 1955), anoxic encephalopathy (Goldberg 1977), brain tumor (Roberts 1968), carbon monoxide poisoning (Bour et al. 1966), and subarachnoid hemorrhage (Roberts and Pankratz 1979). The minimum period of coma required seems to be 2 weeks (Stehman 1959). Children may also develop ectopic bone after prolonged coma (Jacobs 1962, Pryor 1970).

Soft tissue ossification may complicate paralysis due to lesions in lower motor neurons. Stoikovic et al. (1955) discovered this complication in 6 patients out of 1980 who had been admitted with poliomyelitis. It is thus an infrequent complication of poliomyelitis and tends to be restricted to patients who are extensively paralysed (Hansson and Austlid 1955).

Clinical Features

Ectopic bone in paraplegic patients is never found above the level of the paralysis. Many patients have no local symptoms and the bone is discovered as an incidental finding on a radiograph requested for some other purpose. Serial studies indicate that ectopic bone usually becomes radiologically evident at 1 to 4 months after the cord injury (Stover et al. 1975). Some patients, the exact proportion is unknown, develop local symptoms. These consist of warmth, redness and swelling. If the cord lesion is incomplete then pain and tenderness may also be noted. These symptoms may lead to mistaken diagnoses of cellulitis, acute arthritis (Goldberg 1977), superficial thrombophlebitis (Stoikovic et al. 1955, Hassard 1975) or deep venous thrombosis (Ditunno and Venier 1970). Loss of range of motion may accompany these acute signs, or may develop insidiously and suggest contractures or spasticity (Wharton and Morgan 1970). Occasionally, bilateral knee effusions have been noted (Hardy and Dickson 1963, Furman et al. 1970). Severe restriction of joint movement, sufficient to interfere with rehabilitation, was noted in 20 (3%) of 447 traumatic paraplegics in one study (Wharton and Morgan 1970).

Ectopic ossification in paraplegics is usually para-articular and most commonly involves the hip (Fig. 5.1). Less commonly the knee is involved and other sites of involvement are rare (Nath et al. 1978). Of 76 affected paraplegics in the series of Stover et al. (1975), 44 (58%) had multiple areas of ectopic bone and 65 (86%) had hip involvement. Involvement, when bilateral, was usually asymmetric. The impression that ectopic bone is more common in young adult male paraplegics (Wharton and Morgan 1970, Rosin 1975) has not been supported by statistical analysis (Hernandez et al. 1978).

Results of routine laboratory tests, including serum calcium, phosphate, and alkaline phosphatase levels, are usually within normal limits. Increased alkaline

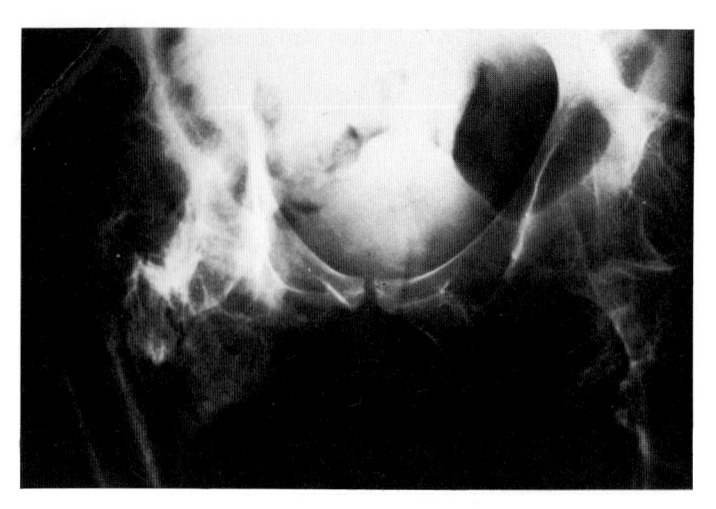

Fig.5.1. Ectopic ossification around the hips due to paraplegia.

phosphatase has been noted in some patients during the period of active ossification and this may aid in identifying patients with ectopic ossification who have clinical findings suggestive of inflammation (Nicholas 1973, Nechwatal 1973). Hsu et al. (1975) could find no correlation between the degree of elevation of alkaline phosphatase and the severity of ectopic ossification, but noted that levels dropped with maturity of the lesion. Increased levels of urinary hydroxyproline during the period of active ossification have been noted by some authors (Benassy and Combelles 1971, Rossier et al. 1973) but this is not invariable (Chantraine 1971). Metabolic studies using ^{45}Ca suggest that there is rapid turnover of newly formed ectopic bone (Chantraine and Minaire 1981).

Ectopic bone in quadriplegics also tends to be para-articular and is only found below the level of paralysis. Hip involvement is commonest, followed by knees, elbows and shoulders (Wharton and Morgan 1970). Paraspinal ossification is uncommon and involvement of the hand has only been reported twice (Lynch et al. 1981, Henderson and Reid 1981). The clinical presentation is similar to that described for paraplegia.

In contrast, the shoulders and the posterior aspect of the elbows are the usual sites of involvement in ectopic ossification secondary to prolonged coma (Fig. 5.2, Mendelson et al. 1975, Mielants et al. 1975). Involvement of the shoulder rarely causes functional impairment and with elbow involvement, pronation–supination may be spared (Roberts and Pankratz 1979). Occasionally the hips or knees may be affected (Money 1972). In the 57 patients described by Garland et al. (1980) with ectopic ossification after head injury, complete ankylosis occurred in 16 joints: 8 elbows, 6 hips and 2 shoulders. Most cases are detected at 50 to 120 days after the onset of the coma (Mendelson et al. 1975).

Para-articular involvement, especially of the knee, hip or shoulder, also occurs in poliomyelitis. Local pain, swelling and reduced range of movement at 6 to 10 weeks after the start of the illness may occur or the bone may be discovered when an x-ray film is taken for some other purpose (Hess 1951, Costello and Brown 1951).

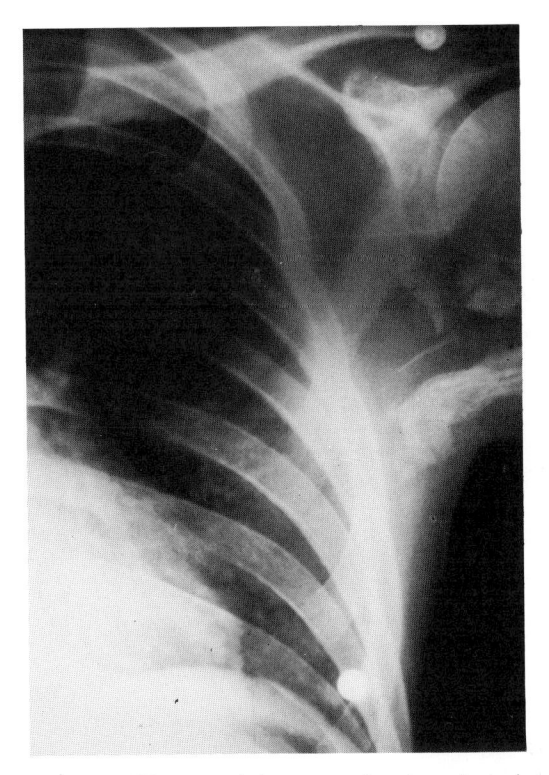

Fig.5.2. Axillary ectopic bone secondary to prolonged coma.

Thus ectopic ossification in these diverse neurological conditions has features in common. Functional immobility of limbs seems to be a key factor in all and the bone which forms tends to be para-articular; to occur at 1 to 4 months after the onset of the period of immobility; and to be usually asymptomatic but occasionally associated with local changes clinically suggestive of inflammation.

Radiology

Initially, there is soft tissue swelling and this is followed by patchy calcification which progresses to the appearance of mature bone (Fig. 5.3, Hsu et al. 1975). The adjacent bone shows no periosteal reaction but the ectopic bone may eventually blend with and obscure its cortex (Greenfield 1980). Ossification may be evident as early as 3 weeks after the cord injury but is usually discovered after 1 to 4 months (Liberson 1953, Stover et al. 1975). Disuse osteoporosis is marked in the paralysed limbs. Routine x-ray films may not show calcification for 7 to 10 days after clinical signs have appeared and in these cases a positive bone scan will aid diagnosis (Muheim et al. 1973, Hsu et al. 1975, Prakash et al. 1978).

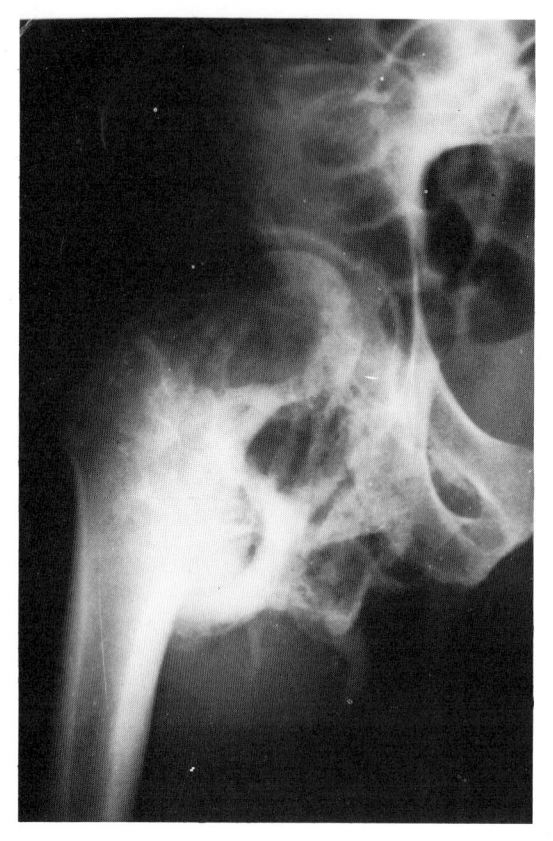

Fig.5.3. Mature ectopic bone in a paraplegic patient.

Pathology

The para-articular ossifications of paraplegics have certain anatomical sites of predilection. These include the anterior inferior iliac spine to the intertrochanteric line, the ischium to the posterior edge of the greater trochanter, the inferior pubic ramus to the lesser trochanter, the peri-diaphyseal region of the femoral shaft and adjacent to the medial femoral condyle (Lodge 1963).

Rossier et al. (1973) have studied the pathological changes in the ossifications associated with paraplegia. They noted initial connective tissue edema and proliferation of fibroblasts. Subsequently, chondrogenesis and osteogenesis became apparent. The initial mineralization involved an amorphous calcium phosphate which was gradually replaced by enlarging hydroxyapatite crystals. This led to lamellar cortico-spongiosal bone, with a thin cortex of tightly latticed spongiosa with occasional Haversian systems. Miller and O'Neill (1949) found a similar appearance in biopsy specimens from 11 patients and concluded that the ectopic bone was histologically indistinguishable from normal bone. Further, these ectopic ossifications have the same x-ray diffraction pattern as the apatite crystals of normal bone (Kewalramani 1977). The histopathology of ectopic bone secondary to other neurological lesions has been less well studied and most specimens have been obtained late in the disease course at the time of attempted surgical mobilization. These specimens invariably revealed mature lamellar bone often with active marrow (Lorber 1953, Radt 1970, Mendleson et al. 1975, Goldberg 1977).

Pathogenesis

Functional immobility seems to be the common factor in these diverse neurological conditions and this has been stressed by several authors (Stehman 1959, Mielants et al. 1975). Early ideas that urinary tract infection, hypoproteinemia, edema or decubitus ulcers might be responsible have been discredited (Hardy and Dickson 1963, Lodge 1963, Wright et al. 1965). Hassard (1975) did note an association between unilateral ossification and an ulcer of the same side, but found that the ectopic bone preceded the ulcer and favored it by reducing the mobility of that side. Déjérine et al. (1919) believed that irritability of the interomediolateral columns of the spinal cord, periarticular edema and inflammation might lead to lowered connective tissue resistance sufficient to activate osteogenic precursors. Rossier et al. (1973) supported the importance of local changes in tissue environment and noted increased vascularity of the paralysed limbs, especially in the region of the hip, on angiograms. Early attempts to isolate a local tissue factor with osteogenic activity were, however, unsuccessful (Curran and Collins 1957). Thus the mechanism by which the mesenchymal cells of the connective tissue with osteogenic potential (the inducible osteogenic precursor cells: see p. 112) are activated in neurological conditions is unknown. Local changes may also influence fracture healing since long-bone fractures in paraplegics and patients suffering from severe head injuries heal rapidly with production of excessive callus (McMaster and Stauffer 1975).

The role of trauma has been disputed and this has led to conflicting proposals about management. Miller and O'Neill (1949) suggested that trauma during well-meaning physiotherapy might be a prime causative factor. However, Wharton and Morgan (1970) could find no difference in the incidence of ectopic bone between their patients who received early, and those who received late, passive range of motion exercises. Furthermore, soft tissue ossification is rare in hemiplegic patients with gleno-humeral subluxation or after intensive physiotherapy (Mendleson et al. 1975). Wright et al. (1965) also pointed out the lack of distal extremity involvement which might be expected if microtrauma were an important pathogenic factor.

Whatever the exact stimulus for osteogenesis, there is undoubtedly an individual predisposition since only a proportion of those at risk develop this complication.

Minaire et al. (1978) found the histocompatibility antigen B18 was present in 11 (26%) of 43 paraplegics with soft tissue ossification but none of 25 paraplegics without this complication. This finding has not been confirmed, however, by two other, albeit smaller, studies (Weiss et al. 1979, Hunter et al. 1980). More recently, Larson et al. (1981) tested for B27 in 43 paraplegic patients. This antigen was present in 5 of 21 with ectopic bone but none of the 22 without ($p=0.021$).

Natural History

Unless the neurological lesion is progressive, no new lesions develop beyond 12 months from the onset of paralysis (Heilbrun and Kuhn 1947). Indeed, after cord injury most lesions are apparent before 6 months, and very few either make their appearance between 6 and 12 months or progress after 14 months (Prakash et al. 1978, Sazbon et al. 1981). Once the area of ectopic bone is mature, reactivation of activity does not occur (Radt 1970).

Spontaneous regression of the ectopic bone secondary to neurological lesions has not been reported in adults but in children it may be expected if they make neurological improvement (Lorber 1953, Jacobs 1962, Pryor 1970).

Management

Management may be considered in two sections: the management of established ossifications and their prophylaxis.

The local symptoms of the early ossifying lesions can be dramatically reduced by corticosteroids but there is no evidence that this influences the subsequent progression of ossification (Hassard 1975). Wharton and Morgan (1970) recommend daily passive range of motion exercises, as their patients with early ossification who did not receive such physiotherapy rapidly developed ankylosis. Hsu et al. (1975) also favor physical therapy in the early stages to maintain range of motion. Stover et al. (1975) used early aggressive physiotherapy in several patients with bilateral ossifications and by using one side as a control concluded that this approach was beneficial. The weight of evidence would thus seem to favor the early use of physiotherapy in patients with active ossification.

In the later stages, management depends upon symptoms. Most patients will not require specific therapy for the ectopic bone but those with ankylosis which is interfering with rehabilitation will require the bone to be excised. After traumatic paraplegia, 8%–20% of patients will require surgery for ankylosis (Hardy and Dickson 1963, Stover et al. 1976a). Tibone et al. (1978) have suggested that surgery is indicated if the range of hip movement is less than 50 degrees. Surgery should be deferred until the ectopic bone is mature, as evidenced by a stable radiological appearance, a normal serum alkaline phosphatase level and decreasing isotope uptake on serial bone scans. A delay of 18 to 30 months may be necessary, but earlier surgery invariably results in rapid re-ankylosis (Armstrong-Ressy et al. 1959, Rossier et al. 1973, Tibone et al. 1978). Hsu et al. (1975) met these criteria before removing ectopic bone from the region of the hips in 6 paraplegic patients: in all the range of motions was considerably increased post-operatively; however, by 1 year some loss of range had recurred but was still adequate to allow sitting.

Corticosteroids, antibiotics, anticoagulants, short-wave diathermy, ultrasound, radiotherapy or disodium etidronate are ineffective against established ossifications and do not reduce the incidence of recurrent ossification after surgery (Fleming 1957, Mead et al. 1963, Wharton and Morgan 1970, Stover et al. 1976b).

The successful use of fat transplants by Riska and Michelsson (1979) to inhibit re-ossification after excision of ectopic bone secondary to hip replacement merits evaluation in this situation. Wharton and Morgan (1970) reported a different approach which was successful in 22 patients with hip ankylosis secondary to paraplegia. They forcibly manipulated these paraplegic patients in order to fracture the ectopic bone and then gave physiotherapy to encourage the development of a pseudarthrosis. No patient treated in this way developed re-ankylosis and this line of approach also merits further assessment.

After prolonged coma surgery may be required for bony ankylosis of the elbow. Roberts and Pankratz (1979) reported 9 instances of excision of ectopic bone in this situation. All of their patients had full restoration of function without evidence of recurrence at follow-up of 10 months to 8.7 years. It is probably important that in each of these patients, sufficient neurological function had returned to allow use of the limb post-operatively. Removal of ectopic bone from about the hip in 3 of these patients resulted in rapid re-ankylosis. Garland et al. (1980) had a similar experience, with no recurrence after elbow mobilization but poor results after removal of bone from about the hip. Again fat transplants deserve evaluation in this situation.

Prophylaxis of ectopic bone after neurological lesions has centered around physiotherapy programs and more recently the diphosphonates. Several groups of authors are of the opinion that early passive mobilization and range of motion exercises may help prevent ectopic ossification or at least ankylosis (Abramson 1948, Damanski 1961, Hardy and Dickson 1963, Couvée 1971, Nicholas 1973). Objective data to support this view are, however, not available.

Stover et al. (1976a) reported a double-blind trial of disodium etidronate versus a placebo in a series of 149 paraplegics. The radiological incidence of ectopic ossification was reduced in those on the drug, but upon stopping the drug this difference was lost. Thus it appeared that the diphosphonate delayed mineralization but did not influence the production of bone matrix. One point of criticism of this study was the long delay after the onset of the paraplegia, on average 8 weeks, before starting the drug or placebo. Many patients already had evidence of ectopic ossification at the start of the trial and ideally in any future study of the potential prophylactic agent should be started directly after the neurological lesion has occurred.

References

Abramson AS (1948) Bone disturbances in injuries to the spinal cord and cauda equina (paraplegia). J Bone Joint Surg [Am] 30: 982–987
Armstrong-Ressy CT, Weiss AA, Ebel A (1959) Results of surgical treatment of extraosseous bone in paraplegia. NY State J Med 59: 2548–2553
Benassy J (1966) Ossifications and fracture healing in paraplegia and brain injuries. Proc Annu Clin Spinal Cord Inj Conf 15: 55–70
Benassy J, Combelles F (1971) Ostéomes tentatives thérapeutiques. Ann Med Phys (Paris) 14: 467–475
Blane CE, Perkash I (1981) True heterotopic bone in the paralysed patient. Skeletal Radiol 7: 21–25
Bour H, Tutin M, Pasquier P, Quevanvilliers J (1966) Les paraostéoarthropathies au décours des comas oxycarbonés graves. Sem Hôp Paris 42: 1912–1916
Chantraine A (1971) Clinical investigation of bone metabolism in spinal cord lesions. Paraplegia 8: 253–259

Chantraine A, Minaire P (1981) Para-osteo-arthropathies. A new theory and mode of treatment. Scand J Rehabil Med 13: 31–37

Costello FV, Brown A (1951) Myositis ossificans complicating anterior poliomyelitis. J Bone Joint Surg [Br] 33: 594–597

Couvée LMJ (1971) Heterotopic ossification and the surgical treatment of serious contractures. Paraplegia 9: 89–94

Curran RC, Collins DH (1957) Mucopolysaccharides in fields of intramembranous ossification in man. J Pathol Bacteriol 74: 207–214

Damanski M (1961) Heterotopic ossification in paraplegia: A clinical study. J Bone Joint Surg [Br] 43: 286–299

Déjérine J, Ceillier A (1918) Para-ostéo-arthropathies des paraplégiques par lésion médullaire (étude clinique et radiographique). Ann Med Interne (Paris) 5: 497–535

Déjérine J, Ceillier A, Déjérine Y (1919) Para-ostéo-arthropathies des paraplégiques par lésion médullaire. Rev Neurol (Paris) 34: 399–407

Ditunno JF, Venier LH (1970) Heterotopic ossification presenting as deep vein thrombophlebitis in the paraplegic—a report of two cases. Arch Phys Med Rehabil 51: 719

Drehmann G (1927) Myositis ossificans circumscripta neurotica im Verlaufe der Poliomyelitis anterior acuta. Zentralbl Gesamte Neurol Psychiatr 48: 686

Fleming WC (1957) Preliminary observations on the use of ultrasonics in treatment of soft tissue calcification in paraplegia. Proc Annu Clin Spinal Cord Inj Conf 6: 18–19

Freehafer AA, Yurick R, Mast WA (1966) Para-articular ossification in spinal cord injury. Med Serv J Canada 22: 471–478

Furman R, Nicholas JJ, Jivoff L (1970) Elevation of serum alkaline phosphatase coincident with ectopic bone formation in paraplegic patients. J Bone Joint Surg [Am] 52: 1131–1137

Garland DE, Blum CE, Waters RL (1980) Peri-articular heterotopic ossification in head-injured adults. Incidence and location. J Bone Joint Surg [Am] 62: 1143–1146

Goldberg MA (1977) Heterotopic ossification mimicking acute arthritis after neurological catastrophes. Arch Intern Med 137: 619–621

Greenfield GB (1980) Radiology of bone diseases, 3rd edn. JB Lippincott and Co, Philadelphia Toronto

Hansson KG, Austlid O (1955) Myositis ossificans in poliomyelitis. Two case reports. Arch Phys Med 36: 506–509

Hardy AG, Dickson JW (1963) Pathological ossification in traumatic paraplegia. J Bone Joint Surg [Br] 45: 76–87

Hassard GH (1975) Heterotopic bone formation about the hip and unilateral decubitus ulcers in spinal cord injury. Arch Phys Med Rehabil 56: 355–358

Heilbrun N, Kuhn WG Jr (1947) Erosive bone lesions and soft tissue ossifications associated with spinal cord injuries (paraplegia). Radiology 48: 579–593

Henderson HP, Reid DAC (1981) Para-articular ossification in the hand. Hand 13: 239–245

Hernandez AM, Forner JV, de la Fuente T, Gonzalez C, Miro R (1978) The para-articular ossifications in our paraplegics and tetraplegics: A survey of 704 patients. Paraplegia 16: 272–275

Hess WE (1951) Myositis ossificans occurring in poliomyelitis; report of case. Arch Neurol Psychiatr 66: 606–609

Hoffer MM, Garrett A, Brink J, Perry J, Hale W, Nickel VL (1971) The orthopaedic management of brain-injured children. J Bone Joint Surg [Am] 53: 567–577

Hsu JD, Sakimura I, Stauffer ES (1975) Heterotopic ossification around the hip joint in spinal cord injured patients. Clin Orthop 112: 165–169

Hunter T, Dubo HIC, Hildahl CR, Smith NJ, Schroeder ML (1980) Histocompatibility antigens in patients with spinal cord injury or cerebral damage complicated by heterotopic ossification. Rheumatol Rehabil 19: 97–99

Jacobs P (1962) Reversible ectopic soft tissue ossification following measles encephalomyelitis. Arch Dis Child 37: 90–92

Kewalramani LS (1977) Ectopic ossification. Am J Phys Med 56: 99–121

Larson JM, Michalski JP, Collacott EA, Eltorai D, McCombs CC, Madorsky JB (1981) Increased prevalence of HLA B27 in patients with ectopic ossification following traumatic cord injury. Rheumatol Rehabil 20: 193–197

Liberson M (1953) Soft tissue calcifications in cord lesions. JAMA 152: 1010–1013

Lodge T (1963) Radiology in the management of paraplegia. Clin Radiol 14: 365–380

Lorber J (1953) Ectopic ossification in tuberculous meningitis. Arch Dis Child 28: 98–103

Lynch C, Pont A, Weingarden SI (1981) Heterotopic ossification in the hand of a patient with spinal cord injury. Arch Phys Med Rehabil 62: 291–293

References

McMaster WC, Stauffer ES (1975) The management of long bone fracture in the spinal cord injured patient. Clin Orthop 112: 44–52

Mead S, Cain HD, Kelly RE, Liebgold H (1963) Periarticular calcification in paraplegics: Attempted treatment with disodium edetate. Paraplegia 1: 62–68

Mendelson L, Grosswasser Z, Najenson T, Sandbank U, Solzi P (1975) Periarticular new bone in patients suffering from severe head injuries. Scand J Rehabil Med 7: 141–145

Meyer P (1927) Dystrophische Muskelverkalkung und Vernöcherung (Myositis ossificans neurotica) und 'Kalkmetastasen' der Nieren nach Querschnittsläsion des Rückenmarks. Bruns Beitr Klin Chir 138: 233–254

Mielants H, Vanhove E, de Neels J, Veys E (1975) Clinical survey of, and pathogenetic approach to, para-articular ossifications in long-term coma. Acta Orthop Scand 46: 190–198

Miller LF, O'Neill CJ (1949) Myositis ossificans in paraplegics. J Bone Joint Surg [Am] 31: 283–294

Minaire P, Betuel H, Pilonchery G (1978) Système HLA chez les blessés médullaires atteints de para-ostéo-arthropathies neurogènes. Nouv Presse Med 7: 3044

Money RA (1972) Ectopic para-articular ossification after head injury. Med J Aust 1: 125–127

Muheim G, Donath A, Rossier AB (1973) Serial scintigrams in the course of ectopic bone formation in paraplegic patients. AJR 118: 865–869

Nath M, Cheshire DJE, Vivian JM (1978) Heterotopic ossification in the lumbar region. Report of a case. Clin Orthop 136: 179–181

Nechwatal E (1973) Early recognition of heterotopic calcifications by means of alkaline phosphatase. Paraplegia 11: 79–85

Nicholas JJ (1973) Ectopic bone formation in patients with spinal cord injury. Arch Phys Med Rehabil 54: 354–359

Prakash V, Lin MS, Perkash I (1978) Detection of heterotopic calcification with 99mTc pyrophosphate in spinal cord injury patients. Clin Nucl Med 3: 167-169

Pryor JP (1970) Dystrophic muscle calcification following cerebral damage: Report of three cases. J Neurosurg 32: 353–356

Radt P (1970) Peri-articular ectopic ossification in hemiplegics. Geriatrics 25: 142–157

Riedel B (1883) Demonstration eines durchachtägiges Umhergehen total destruirten Kniegelenkes von einem Patienten mit Stichverletzung des Rückens. Verh Dtsch Gesell Chir 12: 93–96

Riska EB, Michelsson JE (1979) Treatment of para-articular ossification after total hip replacement by excision and use of free fat transplants. Acta Orthop Scand 50: 751–754

Roberts JB, Pankratz DG (1979) The surgical treatment of heterotopic ossification at the elbow following long-term coma. J Bone Joint Surg [Am] 61: 760–763

Roberts PH (1968) Heterotopic ossification complicating paralysis of intracranial origin. J Bone Joint Surg [Br] 50: 70–77

Rosin AJ (1975) Ectopic calcification around joints of paralysed limbs in hemiplegia, diffuse brain damage, and other neurological diseases. Ann Rheum Dis 34: 499–505

Rossier AB, Bussat P, Infante F, Zender R, Courvoisier B, Muheim G, Donath A, Vasey H, Taillard W, Lagier R, Gabbiani G, Baud CA, Pouezat JA, Very JM, Hachen HJ (1973) Current facts on para-osteo-arthropathy (POA). Paraplegia 11: 36–78

Sazbon L, Najenson T, Tartakovsky M, Becker E, Grosswasser Z (1981) Widespread periarticular new-bone formation in long-term comatose patients. J Bone Joint Surg [Br] 63: 120–125

Scher AT (1976) The incidence of ectopic bone formation in post-traumatic paraplegic patients of different racial groups. Paraplegia 14: 202–206

Silver JR (1969) Heterotopic ossification. A clinical study of its possible relationship to trauma. Paraplegia 7: 220–230

Soule AB Jr (1945) Neurogenic ossifying fibromyopathies. A preliminary report. J Neurosurg 2: 485–497

Stehman M (1959) Les calcifications périarticulaires dans les affections neurologiques. Etude comparative des hanches chez 102 patients atteints d'hémisplégie, de sclérose en plaque et de section medullaire. Acta Orthop Belg 25: 207–238

Stoikovic JP, Bonfiglio M, Paul WD (1955) Myositis ossificans complicating poliomyelitis. Arch Phys Med 36: 236–243

Storey G, Tegner WS (1955) Paraplegic para-articular calcification. Ann Rheum Dis 14: 176–182

Stover SL, Hataway CJ, Zieger HE (1975) Heterotopic ossification in spinal cord-injured patients. Arch Phys Med Rehabil 56: 199–204

Stover SL, Hahn HR, Miller JM III (1976a) Disodium etidronate in the prevention of heterotopic ossification following spinal cord injury (preliminary report). Paraplegia 14: 146–156

Stover SL, Niemann KMW, Miller JM III (1976b) Disodium etidronate in the prevention of postoperative recurrence of heterotopic ossification in spinal cord injury patients. J Bone Joint

Surg [Am] 58: 683–688
Tibone J, Sakimura I, Nickel VL, Hsu JD (1978) Heterotopic ossification around the hip in spinal cord-injured patients. A long-term follow-up study. J Bone Joint Surg [Am] 60: 769–775
Weiss S, Grosswasser Z, Ohri A, Mizrachi Y, Orgad S, Efter T, Gazit E (1979) Histocompatibility (HLA) antigens in heterotopic ossification associated with neurological injury. J Rheumatol 6: 88–91
Wharton GW, Morgan TH (1970) Ankylosis in the paralysed patient. J Bone Joint Surg [Am] 52: 105–112
Wright V, Catterall RD, Cook JB (1965) Bone and joint changes in paraplegic men. Ann Rheum Dis 24: 419–431

6 Other Causes of Soft Tissue Ossification

This chapter considers several conditions in which soft tissue ossification can occur. Some are exceedingly rare; others, for example chronic venous insufficiency, are amongst the commonest causes of ectopic ossification. In most, the mechanism by which ectopic bone is stimulated is unknown and so the grouping in this chapter should not be misconstrued as suggesting a common pathogenetic mechanism, as has been implicated in the preceding chapter groupings.

Ossification in the Arthropathies

Soft tissue ossification, generally of ligaments and joint capsules, is a prominent feature in several of the arthropathies. In each, the primary disease process involves inflammation of joints and early symptoms relate to this. In the later stages of each disease, soft tissue ossification may contribute to disability by producing joint ankylosis. This section will only briefly consider the primary arthropathy in each case and will concentrate upon the pathogenesis and pattern of ectopic ossification. Treatment of this group of disorders is directed towards the primary arthropathy and is covered in standard rheumatology texts.

Ankylosing Spondylitis

In white populations ankylosing spondylitis affects 0.5–4/1000 men and 0.05–0.5/1000 women. Onset is usually in early adult life, with low back pain and stiffness, although more peripheral joints, especially the hips, may be involved (Resnick et al. 1976a). There is a marked association with the histocompatibility antigen B27 (HLA B27). Thus 88%–96% of patients with ankylosing spondylitis have this antigen, as compared with a frequency of 7% in the general white population (Brewerton et al. 1973). In recent studies 20% of apparently healthy people of both sexes who were positive for HLA B27 had some clinical features of ankylosing spondylitis. Since spondylitis is diagnosed ten times more frequently in men than women these studies on apparently healthy people suggest that women have a milder disease (Calin and Fries 1975). On average one-half of the offspring of a person with HLA B27 will receive the gene for this antigen and this is thought to account for the observed familial aggregation (Emery and Lawrence 1967).

The sacroiliac joints are invariably involved. Some patients progress to bony ankylosis and the sacroiliac joints may then be represented only by a thin dense line or may disappear completely. In the spine, syndesmophytes are the characteristic finding. These represent ossification in the outer lamellae of the annulus fibrosus and the immediately adjacent connective tissue. They usually occur at the lateral and anterior margins of the vertebral body and, in contrast to osteophytes, depart vertically rather than horizontally. A common end-result is a bamboo spine with universal syndesmophytosis. The posterior interspinous ligaments may ossify and ankylosis of the hips, knees, costovertebral and other joints may also occur. A distinctive appearance is also noted at the sites of muscle attachments, where irregular proliferation of new periosteal bone leads to a whiskery effect (Berens 1971).

Psoriatic Arthropathy

Psoriasis occurs in 1%–3% of the white population and up to 7% of those affected have evidence of arthropathy. Usually the arthropathy is an asymmetrical peripheral polyarthritis often with predominant involvement of the distal interphalangeal joints. Less commonly, spondylitis is found. More than 75% of those with spondylitis are B27-positive; however, if only peripheral arthritis is present, then only 11% are positive (Lambert et al. 1976).

There may be bony ankylosis of interphalangeal joints of the hands or feet. The sacroiliac joints may show unilateral or bilateral, but asymmetrical, involvement. Syndesmophytes may be found. These differ from the syndesmophytes of ankylosing spondylitis in that they are coarse, asymmetrical, arise from the vertebral body rather than its margin and tend to show skipped areas (Killebrew et al. 1973). In addition, fluffy areas of paravertebral ectopic ossification are common in the thoracic and lumbar regions (Sundaram and Patton 1975).

Reiter Syndrome

Reiter syndrome is a disease of young adult males characterized by urethritis, circinate balanitis, arthritis, conjunctivitis and keratodermia blennorrhagicum. HLA B27 is present in 70%–96% of patients and those patients with the antigen usually show sacroiliitis and spinal involvement (Brewerton and James 1975). Many cases are closely related to sexual exposure but a similar disease may follow infection with *Yersinia*, *Salmonella* or *Shigella*. Eighty percent of patients with Reiter syndrome secondary to any of these intestinal infections will be B27-positive.

Periosteal new bone, linear or fluffy, is frequently seen, especially at the calcaneus, metatarsal shafts, phalanges, fibulae and distal tibiae. The sacroiliac joints may be narrowed but are not usually obliterated. Non-marginal syndesmophytes, similar to those seen in psoriasis, may be seen, as may areas of paravertebral ectopic ossification (Martel et al. 1979).

Enteropathic Arthritis

Enteropathic arthritis may complicate ulcerative colitis (20%), or Crohn disease (5%–10%). A migratory, peripheral polyarthritis or ankylosing spondylitis may be seen. In the latter case, the spinal changes are identical to those in primary ankylosing spondylitis. HLA B27 is found in about 75% of patients with spondyloarthritis associated with inflammatory bowel disease. The prevalence of this antigen is not increased in those patients with only peripheral arthritis (Morris et al. 1974).

Osteoarthrosis

Osteoarthrosis is extremely common. Previously normal joints, especially the hips, distal interphalangeal, cervical and lumbar spine show radiographic changes in up to 85% of the population over 70 years of age. Joints which are damaged by other diseases are also prone to develop secondary changes of osteoarthrosis.

Bony protuberances, or osteophytes, at the joint margins are typical, as exemplified by Heberden's nodes. Actual joint ankylosis is rare. Spinal osteophytes usually arise from the anterior and lateral margins of the vertebrae but in contrast to syndesmophytes depart horizontally, although they may later curve and fuse with each other.

Neurotrophic Arthropathy

Neurotrophic arthropathy or Charcot joint represents an extreme progression of osteoarthrosis following a loss of proprioception or pain sensation and leads to total joint disorganization. In the past this was most commonly seen in the knees and ankles of patients with tabes dorsalis but is now more common in the joints of the foot in diabetics and in the shoulders of patients with syringomyelia. Skeletal bone density is usually within normal limits but fracture healing is markedly delayed (Eichenholtz 1966). Radiologically hypertrophic and atrophic forms may be distinguished. In the hypertrophic type a large amount of bony soft tissue debris forms and later fuses into a large dense well-organized bony mass with an integral cortex. This mass may fuse with the adjacent bone. Periosteal new bone may also occur. In the spine osteophytes are marked at multiple levels although skipped areas may be seen. Paraspinal soft tissue masses containing ossific debris are often present, especially in the lumbar and dorsal areas.

Diffuse Idiopathic Skeletal Hyperostosis (DISH)

Although earlier cases had been described (Oppenheimer 1942), DISH was delineated as a distinct entity by Forestier and Rotes-Querol in 1950. A variety of names have been suggested for this disease: ankylosing hyperostosis of the spine, spondylitis ossificans ligamentosa, spondylosis hyperostotica, physiological vertebral ligamentous calcification and generalized juxta-articular ossification of ligaments of the vertebral column (Ott 1953, Smith et al. 1955, Sutro et al. 1956).

The prevalence is unknown and appears to be age-dependent. Blasingame et al. (1981) found a frequency of 12% in elderly individuals. Forestier and Lagier (1971) studied 245 patients with DISH and noted a slight excess of males and that most were over 50 years of age. Obesity and diabetes mellitus were common accompaniments. The vast majority of patients were asymptomatic but an occasional patient had back pain or stiffness.

Radiographs reveal characteristic exuberant flowing ossification along the anterolateral aspect of vertebrae (Fig. 6.1), especially in the thoracic region, and large pointed excrescences at the vertebral body–intervertebral disc junction in the cervical and lumbar spine. There is also a high incidence of ossification of the sacrotuberous and iliolumbar ligaments and of bony outgrowths at sites of ligamentous attachment in the pelvis, calcaneus, tarsus, ulnar olecranon and patella. These periosteal changes are identical in both site and appearance to those seen in ankylosing spondylitis (Resnick et al. 1976b).

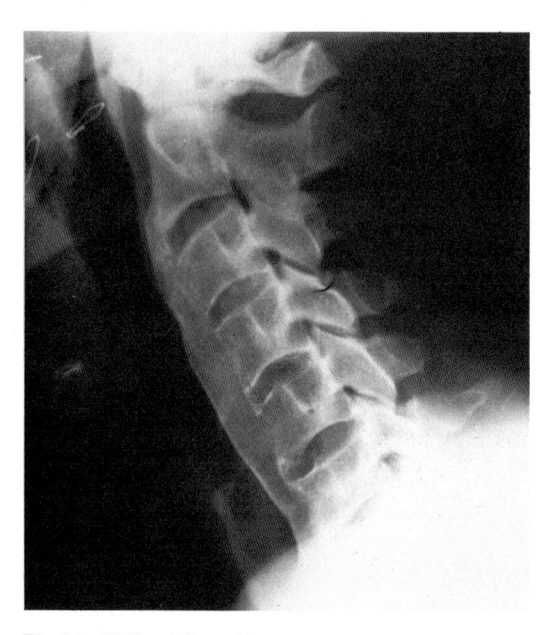

Fig.6.1. Diffuse idiopathic skeletal hyperostosis.

The cause of DISH is unknown. An association with HLA B27 has been reported by Shapiro et al. (1976): 16 (34%) of 47 whites with DISH were B27-positive ($p<0.001$). This association has not, however, been confirmed in other studies (Perry et al. 1979).

Many of the arthropathies in which ectopic ossification is a feature are characterized by an association with HLA B27 and it has been suggested that the HLA gene complex may be linked to genes which are involved in the regulation of osteogenesis. This proposal is discussed in Chap. 9.

Ossification of the Posterior Longitudinal Ligament (OPLL)

Prevalence

In 1960 Tsukimoto presented an autopsy report of a 47-year-old man with progressive myelopathy caused by an ossified cervical posterior longitudinal bar. Other case reports followed and by 1980 more than 2000 cases had been recorded from Japan (Hashizume 1980). Minagi and Gronner (1969) reported the first affected whites. It has since been described in a variety of ethnic groups but appears to be most common in Japanese where it is found in 0.7%–1.7% of patients presenting with cervical disorders (Onji et al. 1967, Nagashima 1972, Chin and Oon 1979). In Hawaii the prevalence of ossification of the posterior longitudinal ligament (OPLL) on x-ray films of the cervical spine is 0.6% as compared with 0.2% at the Mayo Clinic (Yamauchi 1977, Rappaport and Rovit 1979).

Clinical Features

Most patients are asymptomatic and the condition is discovered when a radiograph of the cervical spine is performed for some other purpose. Generally patients are beyond middle age when OPLL is detected, the numbers of male and female patients are equal and there is no familial tendency. Symptoms of cord compression are frequent when the sagittal diameter of the cervical spine is reduced to less than 60% of normal (Sakou et al. 1979). Gait disturbance due to spasticity and tingling or numbness in the fingertips are common early symptoms, but the neurological findings are quite variable (Onji et al. 1967). Occasionally, sudden quadriplegia may occur after minor neck trauma (Becker et al. 1979).

Serum calcium, phosphate and alkaline phosphatase levels, and erythrocyte sedimentation rate are within normal limits.

Radiology

Ossification of the posterior longitudinal ligament is best seen on a lateral view of the cervical spine. Involvement is commonest at C-4 and C-5 but may extend throughout the cervical spine, with or without interruption at each disc. Hirabayashi et al. (1981) suggested a classification into segmental, continuous, mixed and other types. Sagittal thickness varies from 1 to 8 mm and is maximal in the midline. Similar ossification may be found in the thoracic and lumbar regions in 53%–79% of patients (Terayama 1976). Myelography will confirm cord compression and computerized tomography may be useful to delineate the extent of the lesion prior to surgery (Yamamoto et al. 1979).

Pathology

The posterior longitudinal ligament extends within the spinal canal from the body of the axis to the sacrum. The midline portion of this ligament connects continuously with the vertebral bodies and intervertebral discs by fibrous tissue. The lateral portions connect only with the upper and lower margins of vertebral bodies. Ossification starts in the fibrously connected portion. Histology varies from disorganized calcification to true bone which may include marrow (Onji et al. 1967, Hirabayashi et al. 1981). The area of ossification is covered with a thin layer of fibrous tissue which is believed to represent the remainder of the ligament.

Pathogenesis

As yet the factor which causes OPLL is unknown. The high prevalence in Japanese may be genetic or represent a common environmental factor. Detailed family surveys and histocompatibility testing of affected individuals may be worthwhile.

Fluorosis will cause extensive calcification, but not ossification, of the posterior longitudinal ligament (Singh et al. 1962).

Natural History

The natural history has not been clearly delineated. Hirabayashi et al. (1981) noted progression of the lesion in 16% of patients who were managed conservatively.

Management

No treatment is required if the patient is asymptomatic. Patients with cord compression require decompression and for details of the relative merits of anterior versus posterior approach the reader is referred to Onji et al. (1967), Sakou et al. (1979) and Hirabayashi et al. (1981).

Hirabayashi et al. (1981) reported the results of decompression in 53 patients: the recovery rate was 70%. Post-operative progression occurred in 75% of those with continuous and mixed types but was rare with the segmental type. Fortunately, progression was less marked than the original lesion in each case and no patient required further surgery.

Bridging of Lumbar Transverse Processes

Yoslow and Becker (1968) found 24 reported cases of bridging of lumbar transverse processes to which they added 3 of their own. Patients are usually asymptomatic but may occasionally have local pain or stiffness. The lumbar region is typically involved and bridges may be single or multiple (Fig. 6.2). The involved transverse processes may be deformed and the actual bridge is of variable size and shape. Occasionally it may develop a pseudarthrosis.

One-half of the reported patients had a history of local trauma but the proponents of a congenital etiology gain some support by the frequently

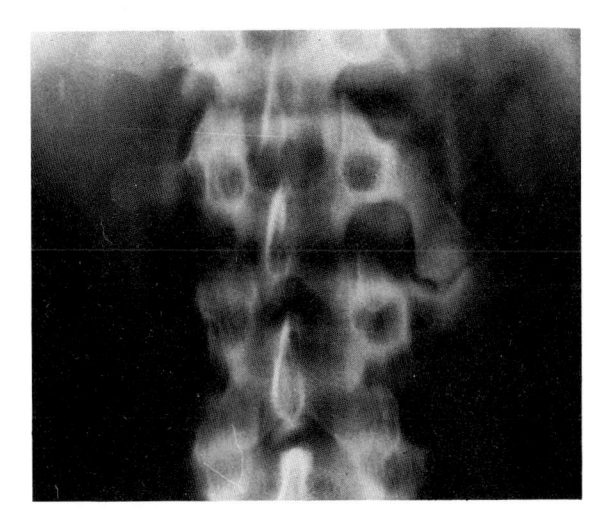

Fig.6.2. Bridging of lumbar transverse processes.

associated findings of rudimentary lumbar ribs, spina bifida occulta, lumbarization of S-1 or sacralization of L-5.

If the patient is symptomatic excision is indicated.

Ossification in Surgical Incisions

Prevalence

Ossification in an upper abdominal incision was first described by Ashkanazy in 1900, and in an infra-umbilical scar by Bernasconi in 1911. Pearson and Clark found 44 case reports up to 1978 and 41 of these patients were males. Eidelman and Waron (1973) noted this complication in 5 cases out of 1600 abdominal operations. However, since many of the patients are asymptomatic the actual incidence may be higher and Mebius (1924) found varying degrees of bone formation in 3 of 31 laparotomy scars which he examined histologically.

Clinical Features

Seventy percent of reports concerned vertical supra-umbilical abdominal scars and surprisingly ossification has never been recorded in a transverse abdominal scar. It may occasionally be a complication of surgery at other sites: radical mastectomy (Fisher 1982) or radical neck dissection (Shugar et al. 1981). White and Hernandez (1980) discovered local calcification after thoracotomy in 4 of 54 neonates. Patients are usually middle-aged or elderly males and although ossification may be evident as early as 14 days after the operation (Lehrman et al. 1962), most present at 3 to 6 months (Marteinsson and Musgrove 1975). Many are asymptomatic and the condition is detected during routine examination of the scar. If symptoms occur then characteristically there is pain on position change due to pressure of the heterotopic bone on neighboring structures (Katz and Levine 1960). The bony bar is palpable in the scar and if the original surgery was for malignant disease, secondary deposits may be suspected.

Radiology

Typically a rib-like piece of lamellar bone is evident on radiographs (Figs. 6.3 and 6.4). The 99m technetium pyrophosphate bone scan may show increased activity in the scar before calcification is evident upon the x-ray film (Pearson and Clark 1978).

Pathology

In midline scars the ectopic bone occurs between the peritoneum and overlying fascia and is attached to the latter (Orava et al. 1980). Ectopic bone in upper abdominal scars commonly has an attachment to the xiphisternum. In paramedian incisions the bone lies between the anterior fascia and the rectus muscle (Eidelman and Waron 1973). Histology in each case has revealed normal cancellous bone (Apostolidis et al. 1981).

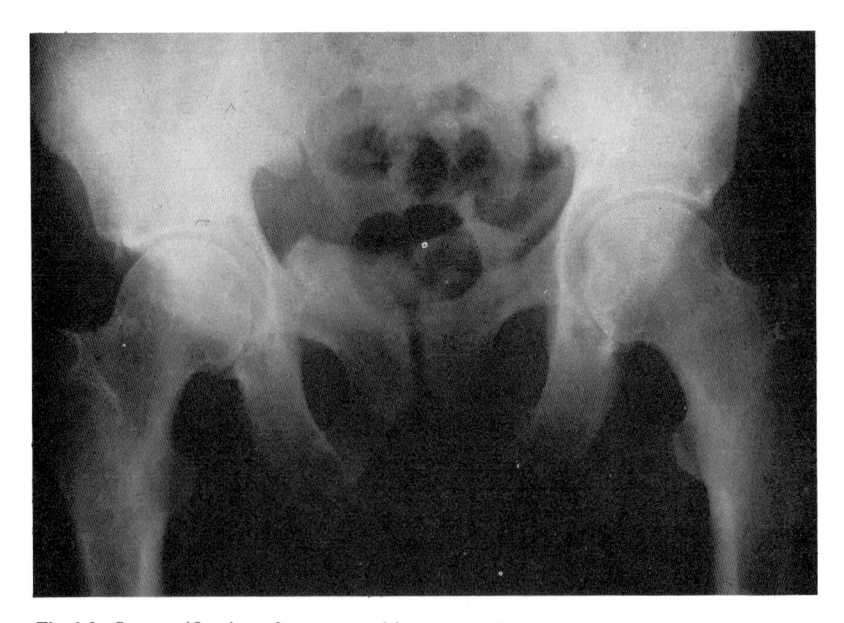

Fig.6.3. Scar ossification after suprapubic prostatectomy.

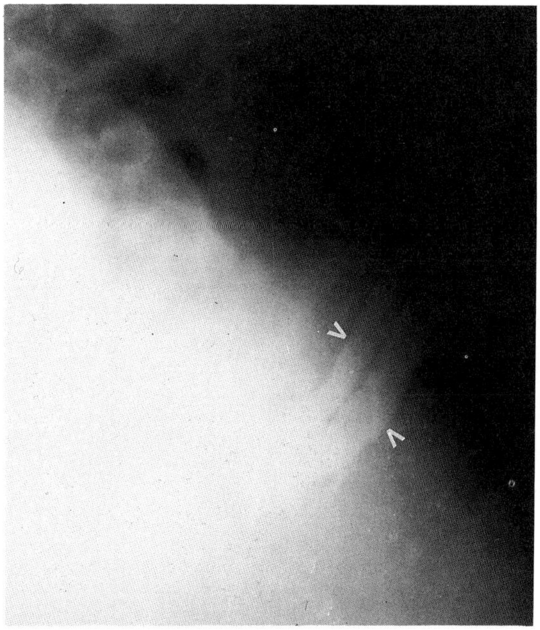

Fig. 6.4. Scar ossification (arrowed) after suprapubic prostatectomy: lateral view (same patient as Fig. 6.3).

Pathogenesis

Scar ossification is not related to preceding wound infection or type of suture material (Orava et al. 1980). Watkins (1964) believed that xiphoid or pubic injury allowed seeding of cells with osteogenic potential but not all cases have attachment to these areas. The theory that induction might be due to implantation of gastric or other mucosa at the time of operation, as proposed by Lehrman et al. (1962), could not account for the cases which have occurred when the visceral mucosa had not been exposed. Local activation of mesenchymal cells is again likely although the mechanism of induction is unknown (Wong and Loewenthal 1975). In addition, only a proportion of those at risk develop this complication, which suggests an individual predisposition. In this context, the report of brothers who both developed ossification in upper midline scars might suggest that this predisposition is inherited (Tama 1966).

Natural History

The natural history is not known; occasionally the ectopic bone has spontaneously disappeared (Marteinsson and Musgrove 1975).

Management

If the patient is symptomatic, excision is indicated. Recurrence post-excision appears to be exceptional (Jaballas and Cogbill 1967, Orava et al. 1980). Irradiation is neither effective nor necessary (Pearson and Clark 1978).

Ossification in Chronic Venous Insufficiency

Prevalence

Lippmann (1957) deserves credit for providing the definitive description of ossification in chronic venous insufficiency. Lippmann and Goldwin (1960) detected subcutaneous ossification in the legs of 60 out of 600 patients who were attending their clinics with chronic venous insufficiency. This prevalence of 10% may even be an underestimate since only those patients with suggestive findings on palpation were radiographed. This complication is undoubtedly under-diagnosed (Condon and Harkins 1963).

Clinical Features

All reported cases are post-menopausal females with long-standing chronic venous insufficiency. Up to 90% have a history of recurrent skin ulceration and this should always suggest the presence of ectopic bone. Obesity and fungal foot infection were also common features in the patients of Lippmann and Goldwin (1960). The subcutaneous bone is readily palpable as hard nodules and plaques of variable size. These may be mobile or be adherent to the skin or deeper structures (Lippmann 1957). The medial aspect of the lower third of the leg is the most common site.

Serum calcium, phosphate and alkaline phosphatase levels are within normal limits.

Radiology

The radiographic appearance is variable and in the early stages recognition may be difficult. Fine granular densities appear initially; later oval specks of increased density, often with a lucent center, are seen. Finally cords and sheets of bone form a honeycomb pattern and the entire leg may be encased (Fig. 6.5, Cohen 1965). These changes are restricted to the legs and are not seen in the feet, arms or trunk (Lippmann and Goldwin 1960). Periosteal new bone, especially of the fibula, may be seen in up to 60% of patients but does not correlate with the amount or distribution of the subcutaneous bone.

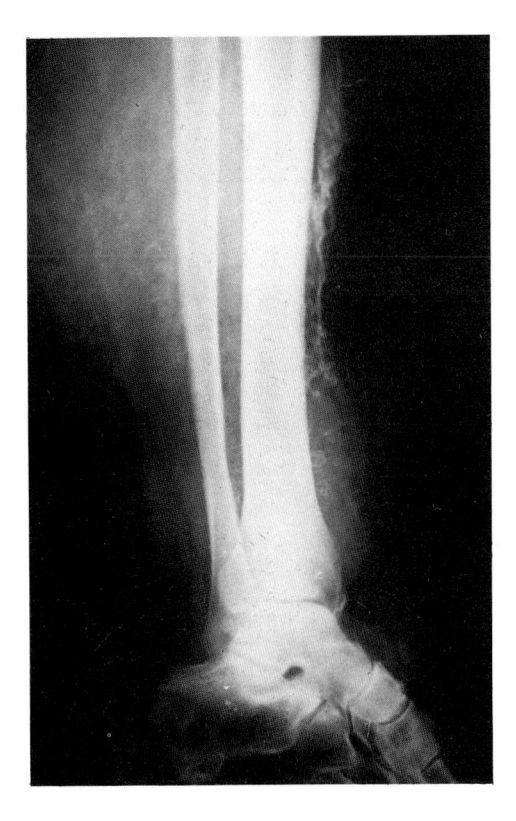

Fig.6.5. Subcutaneous ossification in chronic venous insufficiency.

Pathology

Ossification occurs in the subcutaneous tissue. The overlying skin, underlying muscle, veins themselves and fasciae are spared. Histology reveals cancellous bone in plates or rings at the center of which lie fat cells. Occasionally bone marrow is evident. There is no evidence of fat necrosis (Lippmann 1957).

Pathogenesis

The high incidence of recurrent ulcers in patients with subcutaneous ossification is thought to be secondary to the difficulty of controlling edema in the presence of subcutaneous bone (Lippmann and Goldwin 1960). Lippmann (1957) favored metaplasia of local connective tissue cells to osteoblasts under the environmental changes produced by venous stagnation. It is curious in this condition that bone is restricted to the subcutaneous connective tissue, for although inducible osteogenic precursor cells occur in all connective tissues they are most abundant in muscle connective tissue (see p. 109).

Natural History

The natural history is not known. Lippmann (1957) did not detect any change in the ossifications of several of his patients who were followed for 1 to 5 years.

Management

Surgical removal of ectopic bone is indicated for recurrent ulcers not controlled by continuous elastic support and conservative leg care. The results of excision were excellent in Lippmann's patients: all had permanent healing and none developed re-ossification at the operation site.

Hypoparathyroidism

Prevalence

Soft tissue ossification may complicate hypoparathyroidism of any cause. The prevalence and distribution of ossification, however, seems to depend upon the cause. Most case reports have concerned ectopic ossification in pseudohypoparathyroidism or pseudo-pseudohypoparathyroidism. Steinbach and Young (1966) reviewed the literature and found 57 cases of the former and 20 of the latter: in these ectopic calcification or ossification was present in 33 and 8 respectively. Only occasional patients have been described with ectopic ossification secondary to idiopathic hypoparathyroidism or post-thyroidectomy hypoparathyroidism (Salvesen and Böe 1953, Gibberd 1965, Maclean et al. 1966, Chaykin et al. 1969, Adams and Davies 1977).

Clinical Features

Pseudohypoparathyroidism is inherited and thus other family members may be affected. Formerly, X-linked dominant inheritance was favored, but recent evidence supports autosomal inheritance in at least some cases (V. A. McKusick 1982, personal communication). Patients have short stature, reduced intelligence, rounded facies and shortened metacarpals, especially the fourth and fifth. Chronic hypocalcemia and hyperphosphatemia lead to tetany, cataracts, nail dystrophy and metastatic calcification. A patient with pseudo-pseudohypoparathyroidism has the same physical features but lacks the biochemical abnormalities. As both may occur in the same pedigree, pseudo-pseudohypoparathyroidism is believed to represent a latent phase of pseudohypoparathyroidism. Ectopic ossification in either, generally occurs in the skin. Nodules of bone may be present at birth, or only appear in later childhood. The scalp, hands and feet are most commonly involved (Steinbach and Young 1966, Barranco 1971).

In the other forms of hypoparathyroidism symptoms reflect the biochemical abnormality and, in contrast to pseudohypoparathyroidism, when ectopic ossification occurs it tends to involve ligaments and tendons, especially those of the spine. This may result in marked stiffness of the affected parts.

Radiology

In pseudohypoparathyroidism there is, in addition to the nodules of bone in the dermis, shortening of metacarpals and metastatic calcification.

In hypoparathyroidism due to other causes extensive ossification of ligaments may be seen. Adams and Davies (1977) described a 62-year-old male with idiopathic hypoparathyroidism who had almost complete spinal ankylosis, in addition to ossification of the following structures: sacrospinous, sacrotuberous and iliolumbar ligaments; interosseous membranes of the forearms; medial ligaments of both elbows; triceps and psoas insertions; left patellar ligament and the left Achilles tendon (Fig. 6.6). Periosteal new bone may be seen along the pubic rami, at the ischial tuberosities, at the edges of the vertebral bodies and at the acetabular margins (Buscher 1948). The sacroiliac joints are unaffected and this helps to distinguish the spinal changes from those of ankylosing spondylitis (Chaykin et al. 1969).

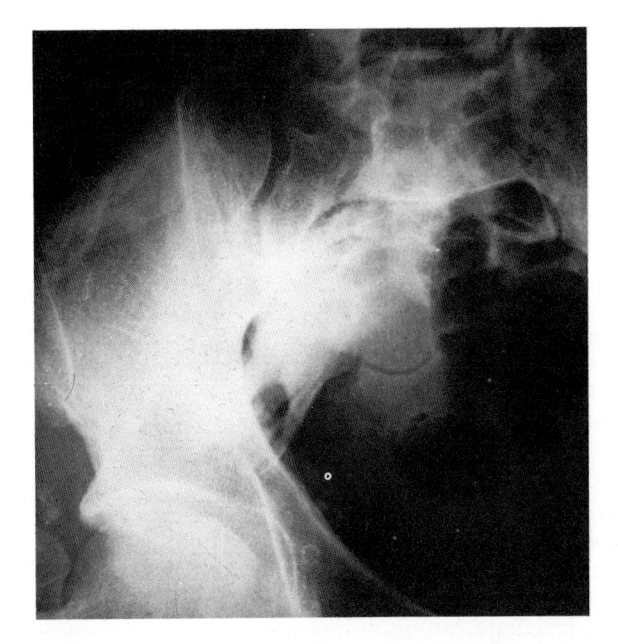

Fig.6.6. Ossification of sacrotuberous ligament in hypoparathyroidism.

Pathology

In pseudohypoparathyroidism the skin ossification is usually subcutaneous, although rarely intracutaneous ossification has been described (Eyre and Reed 1971). Histopathology reveals typical lamellar bone. No pathological studies have been published on the ectopic ossifications in other forms of hypoparathyroidism.

Pathogenesis

The pathogenesis of the ectopic bone in hypoparathyroidism is unknown. Hyperphosphatemia may result in metastatic calcification but not ossification. Furthermore, ectopic bone in pseudo-pseudohypoparathyroidism occurs despite normal biochemistry (Piesowicz 1965). The reason for the different distribution of ectopic ossification between pseudohypoparathyroidism and other causes of hypoparathyroidism is not known. The patient with ectopic bone and idiopathic hypoparathyroidism reported by Gibberd (1965) had a brother who was affected with ankylosing spondylitis. This raises the, as yet unexplored, possibility that histocompatibility antigen B27 may be involved in the determination of this complication of hypoparathyroidism.

Natural History

Ligamentous ossification appears to be slowly progressive in hypoparathyroidism (Salvesen and Böe 1953, Chaykin et al. 1969).

Management

Therapy is restricted to correction of the biochemical defect.

Hereditary Hypophosphatemia

Hereditary hypophosphatemia, or vitamin-D-resistant rickets, is inherited as an X-linked dominant trait. The basic defect is believed to include impaired phosphate transport by the kidney and intestine. Affected males have low serum phosphate levels and rickets in childhood. Females have a range of abnormalities from asymptomatic hypophosphatemia to florid rickets. Serum calcium level is usually normal or low-normal and serum alkaline phosphatase level is elevated when active rickets is present.

Radiographs reveal the typical changes of active rickets in childhood and of osteomalacia in the adult. Ligaments and tendons may calcify or even ossify.

Lifespan is normal and treatment with phosphate and vitamin D has been effective in preventing the skeletal complications of this disorder (Glorieux et al. 1972).

Primary Osteoma Cutis

Prevalence

Osteoma cutis was first described by Wilkins in 1858. True bone, as opposed to calcification, in the skin is rare (De Villiers 1967). It may be primary (idiopathic), or secondary to a wide variety of conditions including surgical scars (see p. 93); chronic venous insufficiency (see p. 96); pseudohypoparathyroidism (see p. 98); acne vulgaris (Basler et al. 1977); scleroderma (Pollitzer 1918); dermatomyositis (Talbott et al. 1959); epidermoid or sebaceous cysts (De Villiers 1967); folliculitis (Roth et al. 1963); pyogenic granuloma (Fulton et al. 1980); chondrodermatitis nodularis helicis (Garcia and Silva 1980); and a wide variety of skin tumors and nevi (see p. 43).

By far the majority of cases are secondary and only 26 cases of primary osteoma cutis had been reported up to 1971 (Barranco 1971).

Clinical Features

The forehead, cheeks and chin are the commonest sites for primary osteoma cutis but any area of the skin may be involved (Barranco 1971). Lesions may be single or multiple and vary from pinhead- to palm-sized. They are flesh-coloured to purplish brown and the slightly raised overlying skin may be atrophic or ulcerated, in which case bony particles may be extruded. Lesions are stony-hard on palpation.

Peterson and Mandel (1963) described a mother and son with primary osteoma cutis, but otherwise all cases have been sporadic.

Pathology

Histology reveals normal bone; the dermis and appendages are otherwise normal.

Natural History

The natural history of this condition is unknown.

Management

Treatment is usually unnecessary (Donaldson and Summerly 1962).

Para-articular Ossification in Melorheostosis

Prevalence

Melorheostosis is a rare disorder which is characterized by irregular unilateral cortical thickening, especially of the tubular bones. It was first described by Léri and Joanny in 1922 and by 1968 nearly 200 case reports had been published (Campbell et al. 1968). Morris et al. (1963) mentioned the possibility of para-articular ossification as a rare complication of melorheostosis and there have only been 6 reports of this to date (Morris et al. 1963, Campbell et al. 1968, Simon et al. 1976, Gold and Mirra 1977, Dissing and Zafirovski 1979).

Clinical Features

Melorheostosis is usually asymptomatic, but may produce local pain and swelling. The skin over affected bones sometimes becomes indurated and thickened. Para-articular ossification may result in joint limitation. Although this has only been seen in the same limb as the changes of melorheostosis, the changes do not necessarily coincide: Dissing and Zafirovski (1979) found ectopic ossification about the hip and knee yet the bone changes of melorheostosis were restricted to the talus, second metatarsal and phalanges.

Radiology

The radiological changes are characterized by an irregular cortical thickening and sclerosis which has been likened to the appearance of melted candle wax. Usually it is confined to a single limb or bone and limited to one side of the body. In addition, areas of para-articular bone may be present which are not attached to bone. There is a high uptake of 99m technetium in both the ectopic bone and the areas of melorheostosis (Janousek et al. 1976, Dissing and Zafirovski 1979).

Pathology

The sclerotic strips are composed of mature bone mixed with osteoid and fibrous tissue. Both cartilage and bone may be present in the ectopic ossifications (Gold and Mirra 1977).

Pathogenesis

The pathogenesis is unknown. This disorder, like Ollier disease and the Klippel–Trenaunay–Weber syndrome, is probably not mendelian.

Natural History

Onset is usually during early adulthood and progression is very slow.

Management

Therapy is supportive.

Miscellaneous Causes

There remain a number of conditions which appear to be distinct from any of those described above. Many of these are single case reports and further experience will be necessary in order to decide whether they really are distinct entities.

Localized Progressive Myositis Ossificans

Patients with ossifying tumors may have locally progressive lesions (Chap. 3) but other causes of soft tissue ossification generally do not progress in size after 8 weeks and have stabilized or decreased in size before this time.

Manini and Singh (1967) described a 20-year-old female who had a 3-year history of a growing lump in her left calf. At surgery this was found to arise from the medial head of gastrocnemius. A zonal phenomenon was evident, as in pseudomalignant myositis ossificans (see p. 46), but was reversed so that the central area was lamellar bone with marrow whilst peripherally lay active osteoblasts and loose connective tissue. There was no recurrence after excision and the authors could find no similar case in the literature.

Rosborough (1966) reported a 21-year-old man with an area of ossification in his left arm which had progressed over 12 years. It lay superficial to the triceps and was attached to it. He also had facial asymmetry, aortic stenosis, flexion deformities of his little fingers and fusion of cervical vertebrae.

Farwood et al. (1978) described a 17-year-old Mexican male with a slowly enlarging ossified lesion of the left cheek which had been present since early childhood.

Cramer et al. (1981) described a 17-year-old female who had developed an ossifying left cheek lesion at age 3 months. This was locally recurrent after multiple attempts at removal. She also had hypoplastic distal phalanges and short fourth and fifth metacarpals.

Ejeckam and Ibekwe (1981) reported an 8-year-old Nigerian boy with a 4-month history of a painless progressive lump arising from his upper lip. There was no history of trauma. The lump was excised without recurrence and revealed a zonal pattern similar to that seen in pseudomalignant myositis ossificans.

Middle Ear Ossification

Horowitz (1952) described a 20-year-old female with an 11-year history of intermittent ear discharge. At operation a bony tumor was found in the middle ear which was considered to represent either ossification in exuberant granulation tissue or myositis ossificans of the tensor tympani. This author could find no similar case in the literature.

XYY Syndrome

Price (1969) studied 12 patients with the XYY karyotype and found in 2 ectopic bone beneath the ischial tuberosities close to the origins of the adductor muscles. There was no history of trauma. No similar cases have been published.

Stiff Man Syndrome

Trojaborg et al. (1970) reported a female with symptoms of the stiff man syndrome, ossification of multiple tendons and syndactyly. Stiffness of the neck was first noted at 30 years of age and progressed to involve the limbs. Radiographs at 39 years of age revealed ossification of ligaments throughout the spine, pelvis and limbs. Biopsy confirmed histologically normal bone in these ligaments.

References

Adams JE, Davies M (1977) Paravertebral and peripheral ligamentous ossification: An unusual association of hypoparathyroidism. Postgrad Med J 53: 167–172
Apostolidis NS, Legakis NC, Gregoriadis GC, Androulakakis PA, Romanos AN (1981) Heterotopic bone formation in abdominal operation scars. Report of six cases with review of the literature. Am J Surg 142: 555–559
Askanazy M (1900) Verh Dtsch Ges Pathol 3: 106
Barranco VP (1971) Cutaneous ossification in pseudohypoparathyroidism. Arch Dermatol 104: 643–647
Basler RSW, Watters JH, Taylor WB (1977) Calcifying acne lesions. Int J Dermatol 16: 755–758
Becker DH, Conley FK, Andersen ME (1979) Quadriplegia associated with narrow cervical canal, ligamentous calcification and ankylosing hyperostosis. Surg Neurol 11: 17–19
Berens DL (1971) Roentgen features of ankylosing spondylitis. Clin Orthop 74: 20–33
Bernasconi (1911) Ossification développée dans la cicatrice d'une taille pour prostatectomie suspubienne. Assoc Fr Urol 15: 746–751
Blasingame JP, Resnick D, Coutts RD, Danzig LA (1981) Extensive spinal osteophytosis as a risk factor for heterotopic bone formation after total hip arthroplasty. Clin Orthop 161: 191–197
Brewerton DA, James DCO (1975) The histocompatibility antigen (HLA B27) and disease. Semin Arthritis Rheum 4: 191–207
Brewerton DA, Hart FD, Nicholls A, Caffrey M, James DCO, Sturrock RD (1973) Ankylosing spondylitis and HLA B27. Lancet I: 904–907
Buscher B von (1948) Osteoarthropathia parathyreoipriva scleroticans. Röntgenpraxis 17: 252–258
Calin A, Fries JF (1975) Striking prevalence of ankylosing spondylitis in 'healthy' W27 positive males and females. N Engl J Med 293: 835–839
Campbell CJ, Papademetriou T, Bonfiglio M (1968) Melorheostosis. A report of the clinical,

References

roentgenographic and pathological findings in fourteen cases. J Bone Joint Surg [Am] 50: 1281–1304

Chaykin LB, Frame B, Sigler JW (1969) Spondylitis: A clue to hypoparathyroidism. Ann Intern Med 70: 995–1000

Chin WS, Oon CL (1979) Ossification of the posterior longitudinal ligament of the spine. Br J Radiol 52: 865–869

Cohen S (1965) The case of the petrified legs. Br J Surg 52: 682–684

Condon RE, Harkins HN (1963) Subcutaneous bone formation in chronic venous insufficiency of the legs. Ann Surg 157: 27–32

Cramer SF, Ruehl A, Mandel MA (1981) Fibrodysplasia ossificans progressiva: A distinctive bone-forming lesion of the soft tissue. Cancer 48: 1016–1021

De Villiers DM (1967) Osteosis cutis: A pathological curiosity. S Afr Med J 41: 534–535

Dissing I, Zafirovski G (1979) Peri-articular ossifications associated with melorheostosis Leri. Acta Orthop Scand 50: 717–719

Donaldson EM, Summerly R (1962) Primary osteoma cutis and diaphyseal aclasis. Arch Dermatol 85: 261–265

Eichenholtz SN (1966) Charcot joints. Charles C Thomas, Springfield, Illinois

Eidelman A, Waron M (1973) Heterotopic ossification in abdominal operation scars. Arch Surg 107: 87–88

Ejeckam GC, Ibekwe O (1981) Myositis ossificans masquerading as Burkitt's lymphoma of the maxilla in a Nigerian boy. Trop Geogr Med 33: 197–199

Emery AEH, Lawrence JS (1967) The genetics of ankylosing spondylitis. J Med Genet 4: 239–244

Eyre WG, Reed WB (1971) Albright's hereditary osteodystrophy with cutaneous bone formation. Arch Dermatol 104: 634–642

Farwood VW, Steed DL, Krolls SO (1978) Osteoma cutis: Cutaneous ossification with oral manifestations. Oral Surg 45: 98–103

Fisher MS (1982) Case report 180: Ossified scars in soft tissues. Skeletal Radiol 7: 277–278

Forestier J, Lagier R (1971) Ankylosing hyperostosis of the spine. Clin Orthop 74: 65–83

Forestier J, Rotes-Querol J (1950) Senile ankylosing hyperostosis of the spine. Ann Rheum Dis 9: 321–330

Fulton RA, Smith GD, Thomson J (1980) Bone formation in a cutaneous pyogenic granuloma. Br J Dermatol 102: 351–352

Garcia E, Silva L (1980) Bone formation in chondrodermatitis nodularis helicis. J Dermatol Surg Oncol 6: 582–585

Gibberd FB (1965) Idiopathic hypoparathyroidism with unusual bone changes and spastic paraplegia. Acta Endocrinol (Kbh) 48: 23–30

Glorieux FH, Scriver CR, Reade TM, Goldman H, Rosenborough A (1972) Use of phosphate and vitamin D to prevent dwarfism and rickets in X-linked hypophosphatemia. N Engl J Med 287: 481–487

Gold RH, Mirra JM (1977) Case report 35: Melorheostosis. Skeletal Radiol 2: 57–58

Hashizume Y (1980) Pathological studies on the ossification of the posterior longitudinal ligament (OPLL). Acta Pathol Jpn 30: 255–273

Hirabayashi K, Miyakawa J, Satomi K, Maruyama T, Wakano K (1981) Operative results and postoperative progression of ossification among patients with ossification of cervical posterior longitudinal ligament. Spine 6: 354–364

Horowitz S (1952) Heterotopic ossification in middle ear. J Laryngol Otol 66: 181–186

Jaballas RL, Cogbill CL (1967) Heterotopic bone formation in abdominal scars: Report of three cases. Am Surg 33: 197–201

Janousek J, Preston DF, Martin NL, Robinson RG (1976) Bone scan in melorheostosis. J Nucl Med 17: 1106–1108

Katz I, Levine M (1960) Bone formation in laparotomy scars. Roentgen findings. AJR 84: 248–261

Killebrew K, Gold RH, Sholkoff SD (1973) Psoriatic spondylitis. Radiology 108: 9–16

Lambert JR, Wright V, Rajah SM, Moll JMH (1976) Histocompatibility antigens in psoriatic arthritis. Ann Rheum Dis 35: 526–530

Lehrman A, Pratt JH, Parkhill EM (1962) Heterotopic bone in laparotomy scars. Am J Surg 104: 591–596

Léri A, Joanny J (1922) Une affection non-décrite des os hyperostéose en coulée sur toute la longueur d'un membre ou 'melorhéostose'. Bull Soc Méd Hôp Paris 46: 1141–1145

Lippmann HI (1957) Subcutaneous ossification in chronic venous insufficiency—presentation of 23 cases: a preliminary report. Angiology 8: 378–396

Lippmann HI, Goldwin RR (1960) Subcutaneous ossification of the legs in chronic venous

insufficiency. Radiology 74: 279–288
Maclean GD, Main RA, Anderson TE (1966) Connective tissue ossification presenting in the skin. Arch Dermatol 94: 168–174
Manini PS, Singh M (1967) Localized myositis ossificans progressiva. A case report. J Bone Joint Surg [Am] 49: 955–960
Marteinsson BTH, Musgrove JE (1975) Heterotopic bone formation in abdominal incisions. Am J Surg 130: 23–25
Martel W, Braunstein EM, Borlaza G, Good AE, Griffin PE Jr (1979) Radiologic features of Reiter disease. Radiology 132: 1–10
Mebius J (1924) Die formale Genese der Knochenbildung in Bauchnorben. Virchows Arch [Pathol Anat] 248: 252–284
Minagi H, Gronner AT (1969) Calcification of the posterior longitudinal ligament: A cause of cervical myelopathy. AJR 105: 365–369
Morris JM, Samilson RL, Corley CL (1963) Melorheostosis. Review of the literature and report of an interesting case with a nineteen-year follow-up. J Bone Joint Surg [Am] 45: 1191–1206
Morris RI, Metzger AL, Bluestone R, Terasaki DI (1974) HL-A-W27—A useful discriminator in the arthropathies of inflammatory bowel disease. N Engl J Med 290: 1117–1119
Nagashima C (1972) Cervical myelopathy due to ossification of the posterior longitudinal ligament. J Neurosurg 37: 653–660
Onji Y, Akiyama H, Shimomura Y, Ono K, Hukuda S, Mizuno S (1967) Posterior paravertebral ossification causing cervical myelopathy. A report of eighteen cases. J Bone Joint Surg [Am] 49: 1314–1328
Oppenheimer A (1942) Calcification and ossification of vertebral ligaments (spondylitis ossificans ligamentosa): Roentgen study of pathogenesis and clinical significance. Radiology 38: 160–173
Orava S, Tallila E, Larmi TKI (1980) Heterotopic ossification in upper midline abdominal scars. Ann Chir Gynaecol 69: 115–118
Ott VR (1953) Über die spondylosis hyperostotica. Schweiz Med Wochenschr 83: 790–798
Pearson J, Clark OH (1978) Heterotopic calcification in abdominal wounds. Surg Gynecol Obstet 146: 371–374
Perry JD, Wolf H, Festenstein H, Storey GO (1979) Ankylosing hyperostosis: A study of HLA A, B and C antigens. Ann Rheum Dis 38: 72–73
Peterson WC Jr, Mandel SL (1963) Primary osteomas of the skin. Arch Dermatol 87: 626–632
Piesowicz AT (1965) Pseudopseudohypoparathyroidism with osteoma cutis. Proc R Soc Med 58: 126–128
Pollitzer S (1918) Ossification in a case of scleroderma. J Cutan Dis 36: 271–279
Price WH (1969) Heterotopic bone formation in two males with the 47,XYY karyotype. Lancet II: 1134
Rappaport ZH, Rovit R (1979) Ossification of the posterior longitudinal spinal ligament in association with anterior longitudinal ligament ankylosing hyperostosis: Case report. Neurosurgery 4: 175–177
Resnick D, Dwosh IL, Goergen TG, Shapiro RF, Utsinger PD, Wiesner KB, Bryan BL (1976a) Clinical and radiographic abnormalities in ankylosing spondylitis. A comparison of men and women. Radiology 119: 293–297
Resnick D, Linovitz J, Feingold ML (1976b) Postoperative heterotopic ossification in patients with ankylosing hyperostosis of the spine (Forestier's disease). J Rheumatol 3: 313–320
Rosborough D (1966) Ectopic bone formation associated with multiple congenital anomalies. J Bone Joint Surg [Br] 48: 499–503
Roth SI, Stowell RE, Helwig EB (1963) Cutaneous ossification. Report of 120 cases and review of the literature. Arch Pathol 76: 44–54
Sakou T, Miyazaki A, Tomimura K, Maehara T, Frost HM (1979) Ossification of the posterior longitudinal ligament of the cervical spine: Subtotal vertebrectomy as a treatment. Clin Orthop 140: 58–65
Salvesen HA, Böe J (1953) Idiopathic hypoparathyroidism. Acta Endocrinol (Kbh) 14: 214–226
Shapiro RF, Utsinger PD, Wiesner KB, Resnick D, Bryan BL, Castles JJ (1976) The association of HLA-B27 with Forestier's disease (vertebral ankylosing hyperostosis). J Rheumatol 3: 4–8
Shugar MA, Weber AL, Mulvaney TJ (1981) Myositis ossificans following radical neck dissection. Ann Otol Rhinol Laryngol 90: 169–171
Simon L, Blotman F, Caillens J-P, Brousson A, Serre H (1976) Mélorhéostose et pathologie articulaire de la hanche. Rev Rhum Mal Osteoartic 43: 737–741
Singh A, Dass R, Hayreh SS, Jolly SS (1962) Systemic changes in endemic flurosis. J Bone Joint Surg [Br] 44: 806–815
Smith CF, Pugh DG, Polley HF (1955) Physiologic vertebral ligamentous calcification: An aging

process. AJR 74: 1049–1058
Steinbach HL, Young DA (1966) The roentgen appearance of pseudohypoparathyroidism (PH) and pseudo-pseudohypoparathyroidism (PPH). AJR 97: 49–66
Sundaram M, Patton JT (1975) Paravertebral ossification in psoriasis and Reiter's disease. Br J Radiol 48: 628–633
Sutro CJ, Ehrlich DE, Witten M (1956) Generalized juxta-articular ossification of ligaments of the vertebral column and of the ligamentous and tendinous tissues of the extremities (also known as Bechterew's disease, osteophytosis and spondylosis deformans). Bull Hosp Joint Dis 17: 343–357
Talbott JH, Koepf GF, Culver GJ, Terplan K (1959) Dermatomyositis, disseminated calcinosis and metaplastic ossification—clinical studies over a period of 7 years in a female with rheumatoid arthritis. Arthritis Rheum 2: 499–512
Tama L (1966) Heterotopic bone formation in abdominal surgical scars. A report of two cases in brothers. JAMA 197: 219–221
Terayama K (1976) The ossification of the cervical posterior longitudinal ligament. J Jpn Orthop Assoc 50: 415–442
Trojaborg W, Rowland LP, Katz RI, Wheaton EA (1970) Stiff muscles and bony tendons. Trans Am Neurol Assoc 95: 169–172
Tsukimoto H (1960) A case report: Autopsy of syndrome of compression of spinal cord owing to ossification within spinal canal of cervical spine. Arch Jpn Chiropody 29: 1003–1007
Watkins GL (1964) Bone formation in abdominal scars after xiphoidectomy. Arch Surg 89: 731–734
White SJ, Hernandez RJ (1980) Calcification in the soft tissues of the chest after thoracotomy. Skeletal Radiol 5: 109–110
Wilkins M (1858) Über die Verknocherung und Verkalkung der Haut: Inaugural Dissertation. WF Kaestner, Gottingen, Germany, p 18
Wong J, Loewenthal J (1975) Heterotopic bone formation in abdominal scars. Surg Gynecol Obstet 140: 893–895
Yamomoto I, Kageyama N, Nakamura K, Takahashi T (1979) Computed tomography in ossification of the posterior longitudinal ligament in the cervical spine. Surg Neurol 12: 414–418
Yamauchi H (1977) Roentgenographic investigations on the ossification of the cervical posterior longitudinal ligament in the United States of America. Orthop Surg (Jap) 28: 757–765
Yoslow W, Becker MH (1968) Osseous bridges between the transverse processes of the lumbar spine. Report of three cases and review of the literature. J Bone Joint Surg [Am] 50: 513–520

7 Experimental Production of Ectopic Bone

Ectopic osteogenesis has been the subject of intensive investigation and there are three fundamental questions to answer. What conditions can induce ectopic bone? Which cells in the soft tissues have the potential to become osteoblasts? How do these observations correlate with pathological soft tissue ossification in man? The first two questions will be considered in this chapter whilst the third is discussed in Chap. 9.

Traumatic Induction of Bone

The induction of soft tissue ossification by trauma is an obvious starting point since this is one of the commonest forms of ectopic ossification in man. There are many reports of ossification subsequent to mechanical injury to muscles or injection of irritants in a diverse variety of animal species. In 1904 Haga and Fujimura reported ossification in rabbit muscles after hammer blows to their legs. Bone can also be induced in rabbits by injection of irritants such as quinine or 1%–2% calcium chloride (Severi 1933, Heinen et al. 1949, Bridges and Pritchard 1958). More recently, Michelsson et al. (1980) described an experimental model for reproducible induction of soft tissue ossification in rabbits. One leg of each rabbit was given a 5-week course of daily forcible manipulation with intervening immobilization by splinting. By 1 week, the thigh muscles showed partial necrosis and edema. At this stage there was also a polymorphonuclear infiltrate and small extravasations of erythrocytes about capillaries, but no large hematomas. By 2 weeks, muscle necrosis was almost complete, with large areas of resorption and proliferation of granulation tissue. At 5 weeks, calcified bone and cartilage were present in an outer zone with some osteoid in a middle zone and a central area of fibrous and granulation tissue. These histological changes are similar to those found in areas of traumatic muscle ossification in man (see p. 20).

Injury to muscles and tendons in rats can also induce bone. Salah and Pritchard (1969) sectioned the tendoachilles and found cartilage in the repair tissue at 3 weeks and bone by 7 weeks. Similar ossification could be induced by blunt tendon trauma. This ossification, after section or local trauma, would only occur if the tendon was subsequently subjected to the pull of a normally innervated calf muscle.

There appear to be differences amongst species with regard to the susceptibility to induction of ectopic bone by trauma. Rabbits are the most susceptible of the species so far examined, whereas direct mechanical injury to the muscles of a mouse is usually ineffective (Anderson 1976). Further, not all muscles in an animal appear to be equally susceptible to post-traumatic ossification. This is illustrated by the inability of Bertelsen (1944) to induce bone in the rectus femoris muscles of rabbits, despite pinching with forceps and injecting alcoholic extracts of bone. This idea of differential susceptibility at different sites in an individual deserves further investigation since it may account for the characteristic distribution of pathological ectopic ossification in man.

Trauma is thus effective in the induction of soft tissue ossification in experimental animals. The mechanism by which trauma activates local mesenchymal osteogenic precursors is, however, unknown.

Cellular Induction of Bone

In 1917 Neuhof used fascial transplants to repair the bladder of dogs. Bone formed in the transplants in every case. This finding was confirmed by Phemister in 1923 and led to the classic experiments of Huggins (1930, 1931) on the induction of bone by transitional epithelium. Huggins placed autografts of bladder transitional epithelium in the rectus abdominis muscle of dogs, and the host connective tissue formed bone. No bone formed when transitional epithelium was transplanted into liver, kidney, lung or spleen, unless fascia or connective tissue was included in the implant. Only actively growing epithelium was inductively effective, and the induced bone was not self-maintaining, as it persisted only whilst the autograft epithelium was present. Gall bladder epithelium was also shown to have bone-stimulating properties (Huggins and Sammet 1933). These findings have been repeatedly confirmed in dogs and other species (Johnson and McMinn 1956, Bell and Knudtson 1961, Anspach 1964, Marmor 1965, Kagawa 1965, Ioseliani 1972). The histochemical pattern of induced bone is essentially the same as that of normal bone. Lindholm et al. (1973) studied the histological aspects of the bone induced by transitional epithelium in rabbit and rat muscles; they noted that trabecular bone with marrow was seen to develop directly from connective tissue without precursory cartilage formation. This suggests that intramembranous ossification may be the predominant mechanism for bone induction by this technique.

Anderson (1967) then made the important observation that cultured human amniotic cells (FL strain) could induce bone formation when implanted into the skeletal muscles of mice. It was necessary to treat these mice with cortisone or antilymphocyte serum to prevent rejection of the implanted cells. By using thymidine-labelled implanted cells, this group confirmed that host cells were responsible for producing the new bone (Anderson and Coulter 1967). The injected cells proliferated to form discrete colonies which over a period of 3 days became invested by numerous fibroblasts. Cartilage cells and matrix appeared within the fibroblastic zones during the next 2 to 4 days and calcification was evident within 12 days of the injection. Electron microscopy confirmed the normal structure of the induced bone and cartilage and revealed that mineralization was mediated by typical matrix vesicles (see p. 121).

Subsequently it was shown that a variety of established normal and neoplastic cell lines could evoke bone formation whereas primary cell lines could not (Wlodarski 1969, Anderson 1976). The epithelial growth pattern rather than the epithelial origin appears to give these cells their ability to induce bone in the host. The ectopic bone induced by these established cell lines was maintained only as long as the epithelial cells survived; it was then resorbed (Wlodarski et al. 1970). The inductive ability of these various epithelial cell lines will not cross a Millipore filter, and cell-to-cell contact with the receptive cells seems necessary (Anspach 1964, Anderson 1976). Species or generic specificity was not required for bone induction. Intriguingly, when cell lines from different species were used as an inducing graft bone was produced by enchondral ossification whereas with cell lines from the same species bone was predominantly produced by intramembranous ossification (Wlodarski et al. 1971a, b).

These cellular interactions may have an important physiological function. As yet, however, this is unproven and the precise mechanism by which these cells interact is obscure.

Chemical Induction of Bone

Levander, in 1938, managed to induce bone by injecting an alcoholic extract of bone into the muscles of rabbits. Lacroix (1947) and others confirmed this work, and Lacroix thought that a diffusible factor was responsible which he called osteogenin. This work fell out of favor when other investigators reported that in rabbits bone could be induced by injection of alcohol alone and concluded that this represented a non-specific response to injury (Heinen et al. 1949, Hartley and Tanz 1951). Interest in osteogenin continued, however, and has recently regained prominence in the new name of bone morphogenetic protein (BMP), largely as a result of the work of Urist and co-workers (Urist et al. 1970, 1977, 1978). In a variety of animals, this group found that demineralized bone matrix when implanted intramuscularly would induce bone (Urist et al. 1970, Urist and Strates 1971). Implants of polyethylene tubes, Millipore membranes, silicon sponges and other non-biological materials become populated with mesenchymal cells but no bone forms. These observations have been confirmed by other groups (Huggins et al. 1970, Gay and Miller 1978). Ossification is not due to remineralization of the implanted matrix, as this is slowly resorbed.

Reddi and Huggins (1972) have described the sequential histological changes. Polymorphs appear transiently, but by 3 days following implantation of demineralized matrix, mesenchymal cells are the predominant cell type. Chondrogenesis is evident by day 7 and calcification of the new cartilage matrix by day 9. Ossification and the development of bone marrow occur at 2 to 3 weeks. The sequence of appearance of the different types of collagen also mirrors that which is seen at normal sites of skeletal ossification (von der Mark and von der Mark 1977; Table 7.1). Reddi et al. (1977) used immunofluorescence to study collagen types after matrix induction. By day 3, type III collagen is present as a fine network around invading fibroblasts. On days 4 to 6 small amounts of type I collagen are detected and with the onset of chondrogenesis type II collagen appears. This persists until the early stages of bone formation. Vascular invasion of the matrix is accompanied by osteogenesis on day 10. Type I collagen was

Table 7.1. Normal tissue distribution of collagen types.

Collagen type	Distribution
I	Bone, tendon, skin, dentin, fascia, ligament, artery, uterus
II	Cartilage, cornea, vitreous body, retina, notochord
III	Skin, artery, muscle, uterus, lung, liver, gut
IV	Basement membranes
V	Basement membranes

demonstrated in the newly deposited bone matrix on day 17 and thereafter type III collagen was localized as a fibrous array about nests of hemopoietic cells.

Bone morphogenetic protein activity is also present in demineralized dentin (Butler et al. 1977), in mouse osteosarcoma (Amitani et al. 1975) and in human osteosarcoma (Bauer and Urist 1981). Non-osteogenic tumors do not appear to produce this factor (Takaoka et al. 1980) and so it would be worthwhile assessing BMP activity in tumors, either primary or metastatic, which ossify (Chap. 3).

The structure of BMP is not yet known and loss of functional activity during purification procedures has been a problem. It is a polypeptide with a molecular weight of about 4000 daltons and is intimately associated with the matrix collagen fibrils (Urist et al. 1978, 1981). It is a diffusible molecule. This was clearly shown in tissue culture experiments where the bone matrix gelatin, prepared by chemical extraction of soluble non-collagenous proteins, was half-digested with collagenase and placed in diffusion chambers on one side of a cellulose acetate membrane with autologous muscle on the other side. In this avascular system, connective tissue of the muscle septa proliferated and differentiated into cartilage but did not form bone unless the diffusion chamber was placed into a vascularized muscle pouch (Urist et al. 1977, 1978, 1979). The BMP activity of mouse osteosarcoma will also cross a Millipore filter (Amitani and Nakata 1975), but it will not be known whether this and normal bone BMP are identical until the structure of each is known. The physiological role of BMP, if indeed it has one, is not yet understood nor is there as yet any evidence for its involvement in pathological ossification.

Bone matrix is only effective in producing ossification if it is demineralized and BMP activity reduced by irradiation or ultrasound: this has important consequences for graft preparation prior to bone grafting (Bang and Johannessen 1972). Bone morphogenetic protein activity is absent from lathyritic bone (see p. 127). Bone matrix from one species is effective in another species but the amount of bone produced shows species variation. Rabbits are again the most susceptible to matrix-induced bone (Urist et al. 1969).

A number of factors have already been described which can influence bone production in this useful experimental system. Irving et al. (1981) found that elderly rats responded less quickly to implants of bone matrix and did not produce as much ectopic bone as young rats. Endogenous calcitonin is not an essential requirement in this induction, but the amount of bone produced was increased if endogenous calcitonin was present (Thompson and Urist 1970). Koskinen et al. (1972) noted that osteoinduction was boosted by growth hormone in combination with thyrotropin whilst cortisone suppressed osteogenesis. Thompson and Urist (1970) also noted that cortisone inhibited osteogenesis and shifted cells towards the formation of small nests of uncalcified cartilage. Unfortunately, cortisone does not appear to be beneficial in any of the human disorders characterized by ectopic ossification and this emphasizes the caution which must be exercised in trying to apply conclusions from experimental animal models to man.

Other factors which can influence matrix bone induction include: heparin, retinoic acid, insulin, somatostatin and antifibronectin antibodies. Experimental osteoinduction is reduced by systemic heparin or retinoic acid (Chalmers et al. 1975, Desimone and Reddi 1983). Retinoic acid leads to a reduction in mesenchymal cell proliferation and also suppresses maturation into chondroblasts. Mesenchymal cell proliferation in response to matrix is reduced in diabetic rats and this effect is reversed by insulin therapy (Weiss and Reddi 1980). Local injection of somatostatin, the pituitary inhibitor of growth hormone release, will inhibit experimental osteogenesis and this effect is inhibited by the concurrent local injection of insulin (Weiss et al. 1981). Local injection of purified antibodies to rat fibronectin seem to inhibit matrix–mesenchymal cell interaction (Weiss and Reddi 1981).

This experimental system will undoubtedly be useful in the identification of other potentially therapeutic agents which inhibit ectopic osteogenesis and in determining the physiological control mechanisms which prevent ectopic bone formation.

Cells with Osteogenic Potential

In the classic experiments of Huggins, no bone formed after transplantation of transitional epithelium to liver, kidney, lung or spleen (Huggins 1931). Similarly, Anderson (1976) found that bone could not be induced by injecting amniotic fluid cells (FL strain) into liver, kidney, lung, brain or peritoneum, although bone formed readily after injection of this cell line into skeletal muscle. Anderson concluded that the host cells which modulate most readily in response to amniotic cells are the fibroblasts of skeletal muscle. A similar distribution of susceptible tissues has been revealed by attempts at bone induction using decalcified bone matrix. Muscle and fascia regularly permit the induction of bone whereas spleen, liver or kidney do not (Gray and Speak 1979, Ashton et al. 1980).

Spleen, liver and kidney appear to lack cells which can respond to the osteogenic stimulus, since bone will be induced, if, in addition to the inducing agent—whether transitional epithelium, established cell lines or decalcified bone matrix—living fascia or muscle is included in the implant (Huggins 1931, Chalmers et al. 1975, Wlodarski 1978, Gray and Speak 1979). Chalmers et al. (1975), however, noted that bone formation was inhibited when living autologous spleen tissue was implanted along with the inducing agent into normally favorable sites. This suggests that spleen, liver and kidney may, in addition to lacking inducible cells, contain an inhibitor of osteogenesis.

Some sites appear to show differences according to the type of inducing stimulus. Hancox and Wlodarski (1972) found that bone did not form after subcutaneous injection of amniotic cells yet enchondral ossification occurred after subcutaneous implantation of demineralized bone matrix (Reddi and Anderson 1976).

Urist et al. (1969) concluded that the readiness of various tissues to respond to BMP by producing bone was, in descending order: skeletal muscle, dermis, brain, lung, anterior chamber of the eye, testis, pancreas and finally ovary. This and the above experiments give an idea of which tissues contain cells which can respond to inducing agents. Next, the attempts to characterize these cells will be outlined.

Friedenstein and co-workers performed an important series of experiments to discover which cells could respond to the osteogenic influence of transitional epithelium. They placed transitional epithelium in a diffusion chamber along with cells to be tested and implanted the chamber in vivo. Cells from bone marrow, thymus, muscle connective tissue, peritoneal fluid and blood could respond by producing bone (Friedenstein et al. 1967, Friedenstein and Lalykina 1970, 1972).

These osteogenic precursor cells were divisible into two distinct types: the determined and the inducible osteogenic precursor cells. The determined osteogenic precursor cells (DOPC) are found only in the marrow stroma and are thought not to migrate in the blood (Friedenstein, 1973, 1976). They have the characteristics of a stem cell since they are capable of self-replication and of generating differentiated cells. Fibroblastic colonies form readily if marrow is grown in monolayer culture. These colonies, if placed in diffusion chambers and implanted into the peritoneal cavity of an experimental animal, will form viable calcified tissue, both bone and cartilage, within a few weeks (Ashton et al. 1980). Thus bone may be produced by DOPC in the absence of an osteogenic stimulus and once formed is self-perpetuating (Hall 1978, Vaughan 1981). Since DOPC within diffusion chambers may produce bone via either intramembranous or enchondral ossification, Ashton et al. (1980) have raised the possibility that this may represent further cellular heterogeneity amongst the DOPC.

In contrast, the inducible osteogenic precursor cells (IOPC) are present in the connective tissue framework of many tissues other than the marrow and may circulate in the blood. In contradistinction to DOPC, the IOPC will not form bone in the absence of an inducing stimulus and such bone persists only whilst the inducing agent is present (Friedenstein 1968, 1973, Owen 1970). As DOPC appear to be confined to the marrow, it is likely that bone is produced at ectopic sites by osteoblasts which have differentiated from local IOPC or from blood-borne IOPC. This ability of the IOPC to migrate would explain the fact that transitional epithelium can still induce bone at sites after local irradiation with 5000 rads. As yet, the relative contributions of local IOPC and blood-borne IOPC in the differentiation of osteoblasts at ectopic sites are unknown.

The hemopoietic stem cells can also migrate in the blood. Thus, if bone marrow is transplanted subcutaneously, hemopoiesis stops, reticular tissue develops and bone eventually forms from the marrow DOPC. This ectopic bone may then become populated by active hemopoietic cells from the host marrow (Patt and Maloney 1975). If, however, marrow is transplanted subcutaneously in a diffusion chamber, bone forms but does not become vascularized and hemopoiesis does not recur (Friedenstein et al. 1966). Therefore, it is not surprising that ectopic bone, in both experimental animals and human diseases, commonly becomes populated with hemopoietic stem cells from the host marrow (Friedenstein 1973, Wlodarski et al. 1980).

There is thus good evidence for the existence of mesenchymal cells in experimental animals, the IOPC, which can respond to certain stimuli (trauma, contact with certain cell types and BMP) by producing ectopic bone. These cells are found in the connective tissue framework of many tissues and can migrate in the blood. The physiological role of these cells is not known nor is it yet established how far these conclusions from experimental animals apply to man.

References

Amitani K, Nakata Y (1975) Studies on a factor responsible for new bone formation from osteosarcoma in mice. Calcif Tissue Res 17: 139–150
Amitani K, Ono K, Sakamoto Y, Nakata Y (1975) Osteogenic induction by cell-free material from murine osteosarcoma and its cultured cell line. Jpn J Cancer Res 66: 327–329
Anderson HC (1967) Electron microscopic studies of induced cartilage development and calcification. J Cell Biol 35: 81–102
Anderson HC (1976) Osteogenetic epithelial–mesenchymal cell interactions. Clin Orthop 119: 211–224
Anderson HC, Coulter PR (1967) Bone formation induced in mouse thigh by cultured human cells. J Cell Biol 33: 165–177
Anspach WE Jr (1964) Bone formation induced by epithelium of urinary bladder. Arch Surg 89: 446–456
Ashton BA, Allen TD, Howlett CR, Eaglesom CC, Hattori A, Owen M (1980) Formation of bone and cartilage by marrow stromal cells in diffusion chambers in vivo. Clin Orthop 151: 294–307
Bang G, Johannessen JV (1972) The effect of physical treatment on the induction of heterotopic bone formation by demineralised dentin in guinea pigs. J Oral Pathol 1: 231–243
Bauer FCH, Urist MR (1981) Human osteosarcoma-derived soluble bone morphogenetic protein. Clin Orthop 154: 291–295
Bell JW, Knudtson KP (1961) Soft tissue osteogenesis with gall bladder mucosal autografts. Lab Invest 10: 397–410
Bertelsen A (1944) Experimental investigations into post-foetal osteogenesis. Acta Orthop Scand 15: 139–181
Bridges JB, Pritchard JJ (1958) Bone and cartilage induction in the rabbit. J Anat 92: 28–38
Buring K (1975) On the origin of cells in heterotopic bone formation. Clin Orthop 110: 293–301
Butler WT, Mikulski A, Urist MR (1977) Noncollagenous proteins of a rat dentin matrix possessing bone morphogenetic activity. J Dent Res 56: 228–232
Chalmers J, Gray DH, Rush J (1975) Observations on the induction of bone in soft tissues. J Bone Joint Surg [Br] 57: 36–45
Desimone DP, Reddi AH (1983) The influence of vitamin A on matrix induced enchondral bone formation (in press)
Friedenstein AJ (1968) Induction of bone tissue by transitional epithelium. Clin Orthop 59: 21–37
Friedenstein AJ (1973) Determined and inducible osteogenic precursor cells. In: Hard tissue growth, repair and remineralization. Elsevier, New York, pp 169–181 (Ciba Foundation Symposium II)
Friedenstein AJ (1976) Precursor cells of mechanocytes. Int Rev Cytol 47: 327–359
Friedenstein AJ, Lalykina KS (1970) Lymphoid cell populations are competent systems for induced osteogenesis. Calcif Tissue Res [Suppl 4]: 105–106
Friedenstein AJ, Lalykina KS (1972) Thymus cells are inducible to osteogenesis. Eur J Immunol 2: 602–603
Friedenstein AJ, Piatetzky-Shapiro II, Petrakova KV (1966) Osteogenesis in transplants of bone marrow cells. J Embryol Exp Morphol 16: 381–390
Friedenstein AJ, Lalykina KS, Tolmacheva AA (1967) Osteogenic activity of peritoneal fluid cells induced by transitional epithelium. Acta Anat (Basel) 68: 532–549
Gay S, Miller EJ (1978) Collagen in the physiology and pathology of connective tissue. Gustav Fischer, Stuttgart New York
Gray DH, Speak KS (1979) The control of bone induction in soft tissues. Clin Orthop 143: 245–250
Haga [ ], Fujimura [ ] (1904) Ueber Myositis ossificans traumatica (Reit- und Exercirknochen). Arch Klin Chir 72: 64–78
Hall BK (1978) Developmental and cellular skeletal biology. Academic Press, New York San Francisco London
Hancox NM, Wlodarski K (1972) The role of host site in bone induction by transplanted xenogenic epithelial cells. Calcif Tissue Res 8: 258–261
Hartley J, Tanz S (1951) Experimental osteogenesis in rabbit muscle. Arch Surg 63: 845–851

Heinen JH Jr, Dabbs GH, Mason HA (1949) The experimental production of ectopic cartilage and bone in the muscles of rabbits. J Bone Joint Surg [Am] 31: 765–775
Huggins CB (1930) Influence of urinary tract mucosa on the experimental formation of bone. Proc Soc Exp Biol Med 27: 349–351
Huggins CB (1931) The formation of bone under the influence of epithelium of the urinary tract. Arch Surg 22: 377–408
Huggins CB, Sammet JF (1933) Function of the gall bladder epithelium as an osteogenic stimulus, and the physiological differentiation of connective tissue. J Exp Med 58: 393–400
Huggins CB, Wiseman S, Reddi AH (1970) Transformation of fibroblasts by allogenic and xenogenic transplants of demineralised tooth and bone. J Exp Med 132: 1250–1258
Ioseliani DG (1972) The use of tritiated thymidine in the study of bone induction by transitional epithelium. Clin Orthop 88: 183–196
Irving JT, LeBolt SC, Schneider EL (1981) Ectopic bone and ageing. Clin Orthop 154: 249–253
Johnson FR, McMinn RMH (1956) Transitional epithelium and osteogenesis. J Anat 90: 106–116
Kagawa S (1965) Enzyme histochemistry of bone induction by urinary bladder epithelium. J Histochem Cytochem 13: 255–264
Koskinen EVS, Ryöppy SA, Lindholm TS (1972) Osteoinduction and osteogenesis in implants of allogenic bone matrix. Influence of somatotrophin, thyrotrophin and cortisone. Clin Orthop 87: 116–131
Lacroix P (1947) Organisers and the growth of bone. J Bone Joint Surg 29: 292–296
Levander G (1938) A study of bone regeneration. Surg Gynecol Obstet 67: 705–714
Lindholm TS, Hackman R, Lindholm RV (1973) Histodynamics of experimental heterotopic osteogenesis by transitional epithelium. Acta Chir Scand 139: 617–623
Marmor L (1965) Bladder mucosa in osteogenesis. Clin Orthop 40: 82–91
Michelsson J-E, Granroth G, Andersson LC (1980) Myositis ossificans following forcible manipulation of the leg. A rabbit model for studying heterotopic bone formation. J Bone Joint Surg [Am] 62: 811–815
Neuhof H (1917) Fascia transplantation into visceral defects. Surg Gynecol Obstet 24: 383–427
Owen M (1970) The origin of bone cells. Int Rev Cytol 28: 213–238
Patt HM, Maloney MA (1975) Marrow regeneration after local injury. A review. Exp Hematol 3: 135–148
Phemister DB (1923) Ossification in kidney stones attached to the renal pelvis. Ann Surg 78: 239–249
Reddi AH, Anderson WA (1976) Collagenous bone matrix-induced enchondral ossification hemopoiesis. J Cell Biol 69: 557–572
Reddi AH, Huggins CB (1972) Biochemical sequences in the transformation of normal fibroblasts in adolescent rats. Proc Natl Acad Sci USA 69: 1601–1605
Reddi AH, Gay R, Gay S, Miller EJ (1977) Transitions in collagen types during matrix-induced cartilage, bone and bone marrow formation. Proc Natl Acad Sci USA 74: 5589–5592
Salah ED, Pritchard JJ (1969) Heterotopic ossification in the tendo achilles of the rat following crushing and ligation. J Anat 104: 181
Severi R (1933) Produzione sperimentale di cartilagine e di osso in seguito ad iniezioni di un sale di chino. Pathologia 25: 611–619
Takaoka K, Ono K, Amitani K, Kishimoto R, Nakata Y (1980) Solubilization and concentration of a bone-inducing substance from a murine osteosarcoma. Clin Orthop 148: 274–280
Thompson J, Urist MR (1970) Influence of cortisone and calcitonin on bone morphogenesis. Clin Orthop 71: 253–270
Urist MR, Strates BS (1971) Bone morphogenetic protein. J Dent Res 50 [Suppl 6]: 1392–1406
Urist MR, Hay PH, Dubuc F, Buring K (1969) Osteogenetic competence. Clin Orthop 64: 194–220
Urist MR, Jurist JM, Dubuc FL, Strates BS (1970) Quantitation of new bone formation in intramuscular implants of bone matrix in rabbits. Clin Orthop 68: 279–293
Urist MR, Mikulski AJ, Nakagawa M, Yen K (1977) A bone matrix calcification-initiator noncollagenous protein. Am J Physiol 232: C115–C127
Urist MR, Nakagawa M, Nakata N, Nogami H (1978) Experimental myositis ossificans: Cartilage and bone formation in muscle in response to a diffusible bone matrix derived morphogen. Arch Pathol Lab Med 102: 312–316
Urist MR, Granstein R, Nogami H, Svenson L, Murphy R (1979) Transmembrane bone morphogenesis across multiple walled diffusion chambers. New evidence for a diffusible bone morphogenetic property. Arch Surg 112: 612–619
Urist MR, Conover MA, Lietze A, Triffitt JT, Delange R (1981) Partial purification and characterization of bone morphogenetic protein. In: Cohen DV, Talmage RV, Mathews JL (eds), Proceedings of the VIIth International Conference on Calcium Regulating Hormones. Excerpta

Medica, Amsterdam, pp 307–314
Vaughan J (1981) Osteogenesis and haematopoiesis. Lancet II: 133–136
von der Mark K, von der Mark H (1977) The role of three genetically distinct collagen types in enchondral ossification and calcification of cartilage. J Bone Joint Surg [Br] 59: 458–464
Weiss RE, Reddi AH (1980) Influence of experimental diabetes and insulin on matrix-induced cartilage and bone differentiation. Am J Physiol 238: E200–E207
Weiss RE, Reddi AH (1981) Role of fibronectin in collagenous matrix-induced mesenchymal cell proliferation and differentiation in vivo. Exp Cell Res 133: 247–254
Weiss RE, Reddi AH, Nimni ME (1981) Somatostatin can locally inhibit proliferation and differentiation of cartilage and bone precursor cells. Calcif Tissue Int 33: 425–430
Wlodarski K (1969) The inductive properties of epithelial established cell lines. Exp Cell Res 57: 446–448
Wlodarski K (1978) Failure of heterotopic osteogenesis by epithelial mesenchymal cell interactions in xenogeneic transplants in the kidney. Calcif Tissue Res 25: 7–11
Wlodarski K, Hinek A, Ostrowski K (1970) Investigation on cartilage and bone induction in mice grafted with FL and WISH line human amniotic cells. Calcif Tissue Res 5: 70–79
Wlodarski K, Poltorak A, Koziorowska J (1971a) Species specificity of osteogenesis induced by WISH cell line and bone induction by *Vaccinia* virus transformed fibroblasts. Calcif Tissue Res 7: 345–352
Wlodarski K, Poltorak A, Zaleski M, Ostrowski K (1971b) Bone induction evoked in mouse by xenogeneic grafts of the transitional epithelium. Experientia 27: 688–689
Wlodarski K, Jakobisiak M, Janowska-Wieczorek A (1980) Heterotopically induced bone marrow formation: Morphology and transplantation. Exp Hematol 8: 1016–1023

8 Regulation of Osteogenesis

Normally production of bone is restricted to the skeleton. The mechanisms which ensure this are not understood, but insight should be gained by the study of pathological situations in which soft tissue ossification occurs. Similarly, a knowledge of the mechanisms which are concerned with the regulation of normal osteogenesis will no doubt aid understanding of abnormal osteogenesis. In the production of both normal and ectopic bone the initial step is the synthesis of a highly ordered organic matrix. Subsequently this becomes mineralized. Control mechanisms may operate at all stages in this process but are likely to be involved in the initial phases of matrix production. Furthermore, therapy which aims to prevent the formation of ectopic bone needs to prevent this initial matrix synthesis. For these reasons this chapter will concentrate on the factors which can influence the synthetic aspects of bone matrix homeostasis, after briefly considering the origins of osteogenic cells and the normal requirements for ossification.

Origins of Osteogenic Cells

There is general acceptance that bone matrix is produced by osteoblasts. Mineralization follows matrix production but the role of the osteoblast in this process is less well understood (see p. 120). There is also general agreement that osteoblasts are derived from mesenchyme (Bassett 1962). The embryonic mesenchyme is predominantly a mesodermal derivative, with some contribution from the neural crest (Hamilton et al. 1962). It acts as a packing tissue between the other germ layers and initially consists of a network of stellate cells with an intervening jelly-like substance. Mesenchyme of this type is present at birth as Wharton's jelly of the umbilical cord, but the remainder gives rise to a diverse variety of specialized tissues (Table 8.1). The primitive mesenchymal cell can thus differentiate into a large number of different specialized cell types (Table 8.2). The term differentiation as used here means the appearance of intrinsic and irreversible differences amongst strains of cells, whereas modulation is used for the varying and often reversible changes occurring in cells in response to different environments (Weiss 1950).

Current opinion supports the view that osteoblasts and osteoclasts have separate lines of cellular differentiation from the parent mesenchymal cells (Owen

Table 8.1. Mesenchymal derivatives.

Bone	Spleen
Cartilage	Joints
Dentin	Bursae
Myocardium	Tendons
Endocardium, endothelium	Fasciae
Bone marrow, blood cells	Adipose tissue
Smooth muscle	Other connective tissues
Lymph glands, lymphatics	

Table 8.2. Specialized cell types derived from mesenchyme.

Osteoblasts, osteocytes	Histiocytes
Chondrocytes	Smooth muscle cells
Osteoclasts	Endothelial cells
Fibroblasts	Mast cells
Erythrocytes	Melanocytes
Leucocytes	Adipocytes
Megakaryocytes	

1977, Chambers 1978, Loutit and Nisbet 1979, Owen 1980). The osteoclasts are thought to be derived from the hemopoietic stem cells of the marrow, probably via monocytic cells (Buring 1975, Jotereau and Le Douarin 1978, Vaughan, 1981). In contrast, there are two distinct types of osteogenic precursor cell: the determined osteogenic precursor cell (DOPC) and the inducible osteogenic precursor cell (IOPC) (Ashton et al. 1980, Friedenstein 1973, see p. 112). The DOPC are found only in the bone marrow stroma and can differentiate to osteoblasts in the absence of an inducing stimulus (Ashton et al. 1980). The IOPC, in contrast, are present in the connective tissue framework of many tissues and may circulate in the blood. They will only differentiate to osteoblasts in the presence of certain inducing stimuli (Friedenstein 1968, Chap. 7).

Osteoblasts have a limited working lifetime of several weeks (Tonna 1966). Hence, since they do not divide and there is a continued demand for osteogenesis throughout life, there must be a continual differentiation of new osteoblasts from precursor cells (Hall 1970). Under normal circumstances this demand is probably met by the DOPC of the bone marrow; the physiological function of the IOPC is unknown, although they provide a likely source for the osteoblasts which produce ectopic bone. The post-natal existence of cells other than the DOPC and IOPC which can differentiate to osteoblasts is doubted (Owen 1970).

Normal Osteogenesis

Bone is laid down initially in either membrane or cartilage. These processes are well described in standard textbooks of histology and need not be reviewed here. The bones of the face, the skull vault and the clavicles are ossified in membrane whilst all other bones are initially pre-formed in cartilage. Ossification in the clavicles starts during the sixth intra-uterine week and primary ossification centers do not appear in the other bones until 2 or more weeks later. In total there are more than 800 separate centers of ossification in the normal skeleton and one-half of these do not arise until after birth (Arey 1974).

Bone growth occurs both in length and in girth. Stature increases by about 3.5 times between birth and maturity largely as a result of growth in length of the long bones and vertebrae. Although growth plates are present at both ends of all major long bones, growth at one end always exceeds that at the other. The growth plates become ossified and growth of the long bones stops at around 16 years in girls and 18 years in boys. Vertebral growth may, however, continue into the mid-twenties. Growth in girth of bones is accomplished by accretion of periosteal bone.

Remodelling of bone occurs throughout life. During growth in childhood, extensive remodelling is required to maintain the external form of each bone, but even in adult life 3.5% of the total skeleton is being remodelled at any given time (Rasmussen 1968).

Apart from growth and remodelling demands, osteogenesis may also be required for fracture repair. Repair is accomplished by direct osteogenesis from the periosteum, in addition to the appearance of a mass of primitive callus in the medullary cavity which subsequently becomes cartilage then bone. Matrix is evident within a few days after a fracture and mineralization by 1 week later. The bone eventually remodels to near-normal strength and shape.

Osteogenesis in the normal individual is thus confined to the skeleton and is a highly ordered process including: morphogenesis; growth in both length and girth; remodelling; and fracture repair (Table 8.3). The mechanisms which control bone production in each of these four situations are doubtless complex and some factors which may be involved are discussed in the following sections.

Table 8.3. Normal requirements for osteogenesis.

Skeletal morphogenesis
Bone growth in length and girth
Remodelling
Repair of injury

Hormones and Osteogenesis

Several hormones can influence osteogenesis both in vivo and in vitro. Growth hormone was so-named because of its importance in relation to longitudinal growth. Congenital growth hormone deficiency results in retarded growth after late infancy: surprisingly, growth in utero and in early infancy is unaffected. Treatment with exogenous growth hormone will restore a normal growth rate (Tanner et al. 1971). Conversely, an excess of growth hormone prior to the closure of the epiphyses results in accelerated growth and gigantism. Growth hormone produces these effects by enhancing collagen synthesis and cartilage proliferation at the epiphyseal plate without undue acceleration of osseous maturation. This is not a direct effect of growth hormone but is mediated by a group of polypeptides, the somatomedins, which are produced by the liver under the influence of growth hormone. Somatomedin C (partially purified) will increase the rate of bone collagen synthesis in organ culture of rat calvaria (Raisz et al. 1978).

Congenital hypothyroidism has no effect on fetal bone growth or morphogenesis but leads to a severe delay in post-natal longitudinal growth with

..rded and disturbed epiphyseal ossification. In the adult, hypothyroidism has ..tle clinical effect on the skeleton, but bone turnover is markedly reduced (Smith 1979). Hyperthyroidism in children is associated with accelerated growth and osseous maturation; in adults, bone turnover is increased and osteoporosis may result from imbalance between bone resorption and production. These effects of thyroid disease on bone are all reversed by appropriate therapy. Thyroxine appears to control differentiation and maturation of chondrogenic and osteogenic tissues (Riekstniece and Asling 1966).

Although sex hormones are produced in small amounts during childhood, they do not appear to influence growth until puberty (Winter 1978). The growth spurt at puberty depends upon estrogen or testosterone. In girls it is likely that the steadily rising estrogen levels at 8 to 10 years initially stimulate long bone growth and then induce epiphyseal fusion with cessation of growth (Brown et al. 1978). Short (1980) believes that the pubertal increase in testicular testosterone has a similar biphasic action on growth in pubertal males. Precocious onset of puberty in either sex produces accelerated skeletal growth in childhood but final stature is often short because of premature epiphyseal fusion. Conversely, individuals, especially males, with childhood hypogonadism are often tall due to delayed closure of their epiphyses and consequent prolongation of the period of active growth. In adults, deficiency of sex hormones may produce osteoporosis presumably by disturbing the balance between synthesis and resorption. In organ culture testosterone has no direct effect on bone (Raisz et al. 1978).

Excess glucocorticoids interfere with bone growth and with remodelling, which results in osteoporosis. The mechanism of these actions is uncertain and in vitro, glucocorticoids have a complex dual effect with early stimulation followed by inhibition of bone collagen production (Raisz et al. 1978).

Insulin has a similar effect to somatomedins in vitro (Raisz et al. 1978). The significance of this is unknown and may reflect similarities of cell receptor sites, since somatomedin is also capable of binding to insulin receptors on adipocytes, chondrocytes and hepatocytes. Babies of diabetic mothers are likely to be large and it has been suggested that insulin may have an important growth-promoting effect during late fetal development (Persson 1980).

In vivo, increased serum phosphate has been correlated with rapid growth of the skeleton during development and deficiency of phosphate with impaired bone formation (Baylink et al. 1971). Raisz et al. (1978) found that increasing the phosphate concentration of the medium resulted in increased bone collagen formation in organ culture.

Glucagon, prolactin, antidiuretic hormone, parathormone and calcitonin have no proven effects on bone matrix production.

Certain hormones, namely growth hormone, thyroxine, testosterone, estrogen and glucocorticoids, are thus essential prerequisites for normal osteogenesis, but the exact inter-relationships of these hormones in bone matrix homeostasis remain to be clarified.

Alkaline Phosphatase and Osteogenesis

Robison (1923) first described the presence of alkaline phosphatase in ossifying cartilage. This finding has been repeatedly confirmed and in this situation the alkaline phosphatase is found on the cell membranes of hypertrophic cartilage cells and osteoblasts (Ten Cate and Syrbu 1974, Robinson 1979). When an osteoblast becomes an osteocyte its level of alkaline phosphatase falls rapidly and thus this enzyme is a marker of osteogenic activity (Hall 1978). The bone isoenzyme of alkaline phosphatase that is found in the serum is believed to be derived from these cells which are actively concerned with bone production, and its level rises in situations where there is active bone formation, such as growth in childhood or Paget's disease (Fishman and Ghosh 1967). In hypophosphatasia, where there is an inherited reduction in serum and tissue alkaline phosphatase activity, bone mineralization is grossly abnormal (Rathbun et al. 1961). There is thus strong circumstantial evidence that the bone isoenzyme of alkaline phosphatase is involved in the mineralization of bone.

Numerous roles for alkaline phosphatase in osteogenesis were suggested including: production of phosphate by hydrolysis of monophosphoric acid esters (Robison 1923); hydrolysis of pyrophosphate (Fleisch et al. 1966); bone matrix production (Siffert 1951); and collagen degradation (Ten Cate and Syrbu 1974).

Anderson in 1969 made the important discovery of membrane-bound vesicles in ossifying cartilage. These are visible with an electron microscope and more than 30% of the total alkaline phosphatase in a crude homogenate of calcifying cartilage sediments with this matrix vesicle fraction (Anderson 1969). These findings at sites of bone mineralization have been confirmed in man and other species by several groups (Sayegh et al. 1974). The alkaline phosphatase lies on the outer surface of the vesicle membrane and increases in activity as vesicles approach the calcification front (Anderson 1976). These vesicles are believed to be derived from osteoblasts by a process of budding and to act as the initial foci for calcification of bone matrix (Felix and Fleisch 1976, Ornoy et al. 1980). Similar membrane vesicles have also been found in mineralizing dentin; osteosarcoma; experimental ectopic ossifications; and in amorphous calcifications at diverse sites including: aorta, chondrosarcoma, costal and tracheal cartilage (Schajowicz et al. 1974, Bonucci and Dearden 1976, Kim 1976, Anderson 1976). Matrix vesicles thus appear to be the common factor in all tissue mineralization whether this is as bone or as amorphous calcification, but they are not thought to have a direct role in the regulation of the preceding matrix production.

Vitamins and Osteogenesis

Vitamins A and C have established importance in bone matrix homeostasis. Moore et al. (1935) discovered that cattle fed on a diet deficient in vitamin A developed bony overgrowth which led to compression of cranial nerves. These animals appeared to have a failure of remodelling with continued growth, especially on periosteal surfaces. Conversely, in three cases of long-standing vitamin A overdosage in man there was hypercalcemia associated with excessive bone resorption (Frame et al. 1974). In vitro, excess vitamin A leads to a marked disturbance of epiphyseal cartilage growth and extensive bone resorption in fetal mouse bones (Fell and Mellanby 1952). Excess of retinoic acid will also interfere with skeletal morphogenesis in utero. In mice excess vitamin A during the sensitive period of days 11 to 13 of gestation inclusive, results in limb malformations and cleft palate but no retardation of overall fetal growth (Kochar 1977). Weston et al. (1969) suggested that these changes due to excess or deficiency of vitamin A may be related to this vitamin's action in regulating the permeability of lysosomal membranes.

Man, other primates and the guinea pig are the only mammals which are unable to synthesize vitamin C and in which, therefore, dietary deficiency leads to scurvy. In scurvy, there is impaired formation of bone and failure of bone repair after injury even to the extent of a complete failure of osteoid formation. These abnormalities are attributable to impaired formation of matrix and especially to impaired synthesis of collagen. Vitamin C acts as a cofactor to several hydroxylases (prolyl 4-hydroxylase, prolyl 3-hydroxylase, lysyl hydroxylase) which are important in the production of normal collagen. If this hydroxylation is defective an unstable triple helix is produced. Production of unstable collagen by ascorbate-deficient fibroblasts can be demonstrated in vitro (Prockop et al. 1979).

Vitamin D has an undisputed importance in bone mineral homeostasis, but has not yet been shown to have an effect on bone matrix production. There is little evidence that vitamins B, E or K have any effect on the skeleton.

Trace Elements and Osteogenesis

Asling and Hurley (1963) provided an extensive review (326 references) of the evidence that various trace minerals play a role in skeletal homeostasis. They concluded that manganese, zinc, copper and iodine were important in this respect.

Trace elements appear to be important for skeletal morphogenesis. Deficiency of manganese, zinc or copper will induce skeletal malformations in rats (Hurley 1981). In experimental animals maternal manganese deficiency results in a variety of skeletal defects including chondrodystrophy, dysplasia of the proximal tibial epiphysis and defective development of the otic capsule which leads to congenital ataxia. Zinc deficiency is probably also teratogenic in humans (Hambridge et al. 1975, Jameson 1976).

Manganese deficiency will result in stunted skeletal growth in a wide range of mammals and fowl. Some bones are more affected than others and this may lead to disproportion in length and sometimes in thickness. The appendicular skeleton is especially affected: skeletal maturation is delayed, joints may be thickened and bony shafts may be bowed. Histology reveals reduced chondrogenesis at the epiphyseal cartilage plate.

Zinc deficiency has been less well studied, but seems to produce impaired skeletal growth and maturation. Zinc may also influence ectopic ossification. Calhoun et al. (1975) noted an association between the amount of newly formed bone after Achilles tenotomy in rats and the serum zinc level.

Copper deficiency results in mild effects on skeletal growth and maturation but bony deformities develop, including enlarged joints, bowed shafts and increased bone fragility.

Iodine is vital for the synthesis of thyroxine and deficiency produces its adverse effects on the skeleton via hypothyroidism (see p. 119).

Mechanical Stress and Osteogenesis

Walton and Hammond (1938) reported the classic breeding experiment of crossing a Shire horse with a Shetland pony. When the mother was the large Shire the foal was about three times larger than when the mother was the Shetland pony. This maternal effect was due to differences in rate of growth rather than duration of gestation. Similarly, in man the size of a full-term infant correlates with the size of the mother and not the father (Crawley et al. 1955). Uterine constraint is presumably greater in primigravidae and firstborns on average are smaller than later-born children (Castle 1941). Similarly, since uterine constraint is an important factor in the production of congenital postural deformities it is not surprising to find that infants with these deformities tend to be smaller than average.

Activity and muscle strength are important for bone growth, development and the maintenance of bone density. The bone spicules are aligned in the direction of stress of gravitational weight-bearing and of muscle pull. Prolonged muscle weakness in the growing child may lead to less prominence of the trochanters and a valgus deformity of the femoral necks (Smith 1977). Similarly, children who spend their lives horizontal develop high vertebral bodies with narrow disc spaces (Houston 1978). Linear growth is only mildly affected by muscle weakness, with no more than a 5%–10% reduction in linear growth rate after paralysis of a limb. Subperiosteal growth in breadth is, however, more dramatically affected. It has long been known that confinement to bed may result in a marked loss of bone mass and osteoporosis. This will occur with bone disuse of any cause; for example, it is seen in paralysed limbs, in functional disuse secondary to arthritis and in astronauts exposed to weightlessness (Mack et al. 1967, Minaire et al. 1974). Intermittent stress on a bone tends to foster local bone growth; however, sustained pressure may lead to reduced local bone production. The pressure exerted by the growth process is enormous and an estimated 400 kg would be necessary to stop growth completely at a human limb epiphysis (Sinclair 1978).

Mechanical stress is thus an important factor in the regulation of osteogenesis during bone growth with respect to length and breadth and during remodelling.

Yasuda et al. (1955) made the important observation that bone exhibits a stress piezoelectric effect. A piezoelectrical material produces a single electrical pulse of short duration and one polarity on deformation and an equal pulse of opposite polarity on the release from deformation, with no continuous flow of current at any time. In bone, collagen is the generating source but the signal is partially rectified at the mineral–collagen junction, thus producing a net transfer of electricity in one direction. This rectification results in areas of compression stress having a net overall negative charge, whilst areas under tension are positive (Bassett and Becker 1962). These potentials may have a direct local effect on the activity of osteoblasts and thus provide a mechanism for the physiological response of bone remodelling to mechanical stress (Becker 1979).

Electricity and Osteogenesis

Yasuda et al. (1955), in addition to discovering that stress generated electrical potentials in bone (see above), showed that 1 ampere of continuous direct current administered via implanted electrodes for 3 weeks, produced local new bone growth in rabbit femora. Bassett et al. (1964) confirmed these results in dogs and noted that new bone formation was confined to the negative electrode. Similar bone production will occur in man and Spadaro (1977) has reviewed the now extensive literature on this subject. Bone can be stimulated in man either by implanted electrodes or, more conveniently, by the induction of currents by an external varying magnetic field (Bassett et al. 1974).

In amphibians the capacity for limb regeneration is proportional to the current of injury and supplementation of this current results in enhanced limb regeneration (Becker 1961); it will even permit partial limb regeneration in mammals (Becker and Spadaro 1972).

The role of electrical potentials in determining osteogenesis during morphogenesis or growth in man is not yet known but deserves further investigation.

Genes and Osteogenesis

There is general acceptance of the conclusion of Fell (1956) that bones are self-differentiating organs. A bone in organ culture will develop and maintain its characteristic shape in the absence of mechanical or environmental influences. This inherent ability is believed to be under genetic control, though the number of genes involved and their mechanism of action are obscure.

In post-natal life the external form of a bone represents an interplay of genetic and environmental factors: the best understood of the latter is mechanical stress (see p. 123).

Longitudinal growth is also under genetic control. By 1889 Sir Francis Galton had recognized the 'beautiful regularity in the statures of a population' that shows 'small dependence on differences in bringing up' and correlates to mid-parental height. He also noted that offspring of one tall and one short parent are of similar stature to those born of average-sized parents. These findings were consistent with polygenic inheritance, that is of several genes, each at different loci, each with a small but additive influence. These observations and conclusions still hold true today.

Stature is one of the most heritable traits recognized in man. The correlation coefficient for stature in monozygotic twins is 0.95; the average difference in height of monozygotic twins is 2.8 cm versus an average difference of 12 cm for dizygotic twins of the same sex (Bulmer 1970). This correlation of a child's stature to parental stature is evident from 2 years of age (Smith et al. 1976).

There is a wide variability in the normal pace of osseous maturation, especially the timing and intensity of the growth spurt, and in the sequence of the secondary ossification centers. These features also appear to be under polygenic control but have been less well studied than stature (Smith 1977, Fischbein and Nordqvist 1978, Hauspie et al. 1982).

Since genetic factors have such an important role in the regulation of osteogenesis throughout life it is not surprising that skeletal morphogenesis and growth may be aberrant secondary to genetic disease. Already more than 100 single gene mutations are known which can interfere with normal bone formation (Beighton 1977). The mechanism by which these mutant genes interfere with bone production and the function of their normal counterparts are largely unknown. These genetic disorders may have their effect at any stage in the process of bone production (Rimoin 1977, Table 8.4). Elucidation of the pathogenesis of these 'experiments of nature' will probably be an important step in gaining insight into normal skeletal homeostasis.

Table 8.4. Genetic disorders of osteogenesis.

Pathogenesis	Disorder
Abnormal cartilage precursor	Mesomelic dwarfism, achondrogenesis
Defective primary ossification	Osteogenesis imperfecta, hypophosphatasia
Defective secondary ossification	Multiple epiphyseal dysplasia
Defective proliferation of the growth plate	Achondroplasia, metaphyseal chondrodysplasia
Defective modelling	Osteopetrosis, Pyle disease
Premature epiphyseal fusion	Dyschondrosteosis

Cellular Interactions and Osteogenesis

Cellular interactions probably play an important, though as yet poorly understood, role in tissue regulation in the intact organism. The ability of certain cells to stimulate others to become osteoblasts is discussed in Chap. 7 (p. 108) and it seems likely that inhibition of osteogenesis may also be mediated by cell-to-cell contact.

Montgomery and van Orman (1967) made the interesting observation that if frontal sinus obliteration was performed in conjunction with an adipose tissue transplant there was a lack of the usual reactive sclerosis which follows frontal sinus surgery. This inhibition of osteogenic activity by adipose tissue seems to occur even when there is a layer of fibrous tissue between the adipose implant and the existing bony wall. Similarly, Riska and Michelsson (1979) successfully prevented recurrence of ectopic bone, after its excision from the region of the hip, by the use of fat transplants. This effect of adipose tissue may not be restricted to inhibition of osteogenesis, for in both rabbits and humans free fat placed on the spinal dura at the time of laminectomy will prevent epidural scar formation (Kiviluoto 1976, Langenskiöld and Kiviluoto 1976). Tissue interposition between fractured bone ends is believed to be an important cause of non-union and again cellular inhibition may be involved (Altner et al. 1975).

Medications and Osteogenesis

Many medications can interfere with bone production during either morphogenesis or subsequent growth and remodelling. Although many drugs have been incriminated as having an adverse effect on the developing skeleton, only a few have a proven teratogenic effect in man (Table 8.5, Shepard 1976). These adverse effects tend to be non-specific and other organs which are actively developing at the time of exposure may also be malformed. Unfortunately drugs which are teratogenic in experimental animals are not necessarily teratogenic in man and vice versa: this is exemplified by thalidomide, which is teratogenic in man and rabbits but not in rats. For the same reason, findings on the effects of drugs on the post-natal skeleton of experimental animals must be applied with caution to man.

Table 8.5. Proven skeletal teratogens in man.

Drug	Effect
Thalidomide	Limb reduction defects
Warfarin	Chondrodysplasia punctata
Hydantoin	Hypoplasia of distal phalanges
Aminopterin	Mesomelic limb shortening

Few medications, with the exception of corticosteroids, heparin and disodium etidronate, appear to produce adverse clinical effects on the post-natal skeleton in man. Corticosteroids retard longitudinal growth, impair fracture healing and interfere with bone turnover, which leads to osteoporosis. These effects are due to reduced protein synthesis by osteoblasts. Disodium etidronate inhibits mineralization of matrix and may result in widening of the physis and irregular metaphyseal ossification (Wood and Robinson 1976). Osteoporosis has also been a problem after long-term administration of heparin (Griffiths et al. 1965). Heparin's anticoagulant activity is strongly inhibited by vitamin C (Owen et al. 1970) and thus the adverse effect of heparin on bone may be due to interference with vitamin-C-dependent enzymes which are important for matrix production (see p. 121).

Harris et al. (1968) have shown that tetracycline, when given systemically, can severely inhibit ossification in dogs and perfusion studies suggest that this is a direct effect. Kaitila et al. (1970) studied mouse long bones in vitro. At low concentrations of tetracycline, mineralization was prevented; increased concentrations also affected collagen biosynthesis; and a still further increase interfered with DNA synthesis, cell proliferation and general protein synthesis. At therapeutic levels in man, however, there is no evidence for any disturbance of new bone formation.

L-Tetramisole (levamisole), which is used in the treatment of ascariasis, is a stereospecific inhibitor of alkaline phosphatase activity. Fallon et al. (1980) studied its effects on rat tibiae in vitro and found a dose-dependent inhibition of cartilage calcification, but preservation of the structural integrity of matrix vesicles. Adverse clinical effects have not been reported, but might be expected with prolonged or repeated courses of this drug.

Chlorpromazine when given to pregnant rats resulted in delayed ossification in the fetus, as judged by staining with alizarin red (Singh and Padmanabhan 1979).

Indomethacin seriously impairs the healing of femoral fractures in rats (Rø et al. 1976). Ibuprofen, another anti-inflammatory agent, also results in reduced bone production after experimental fractures in rats (Lindholm and Törnkvist 1981). Penicillamine blocks the conversion of soluble to insoluble collagen. Thus penicillamine, ibuprofen and indomethacin might be expected to produce adverse skeletal side-effects in man.

Beta-aminopropionitrile, the toxic component of the sweet pea (*Lathyrus odoratus*), is a strong inhibitor of lysyl oxidase and thus of collagen cross-linking. When given to experimental animals it produces lathyrism, in which there is a marked increase in tissue soluble collagen and reduced bone mineralization (Rosenquist et al. 1977). Several other agents, such as arsenate (Barzell et al. 1971) and alizarin red S (Harris et al. 1964), will also interfere with osteogenesis in experimental animals, but as these are not used as therapeutic agents in man, they are not discussed further.

Other Influences on Osteogenesis

Virtually any disease in a child will interfere with normal growth. Prenatal growth is usually reduced if the child is chromosomally abnormal or has been infected with cytomeglavirus, toxoplasmosis, rubella or syphilis. Maternal cigarette smoking and illnesses such as toxemia, high blood pressure, renal disease and ethanol or opiate abuse, may also adversely influence prenatal growth. After birth, acute infectious illnesses produce transient growth arrest and this is reflected by transverse lines of increased density in the long bones called Harris' or growth arrest lines. Any chronic illness may result in a serious defect of longitudinal growth. This non-specific response of growth to illness accounts for the value of the growth record when assessing the well-being of a child. With successful treatment of the illness, restoration of normal growth is to be expected.

Illness need not be physical to interfere with growth. In some socially deprived, although adequately fed, children growth is absent and so is growth hormone. The reasons for this are not known. These children recover when moved to better surroundings, but do not respond to human growth hormone if left in defective home conditions (Tanner 1972).

Individuals with mental deficiency tend to be shorter than average and there is a crude general correlation between the degree of mental deficiency and shortness of stature (Mosier et al. 1965). Mosier and Jansons (1970) in studies on neonatal rats showed that early irradiation damage to the brain was followed by growth deficiency which could not be explained on an endocrine basis. In these experiments, irradiation was ineffective if unilateral and most effective if the midbrain was involved. These authors suggested the existence of a midbrain center which exerts an influence on growth, independent of growth hormone.

Neural mechanisms may also influence other aspects of osteogenesis. Fractures of long bones in paraplegics and patients with severe head injury heal rapidly with excessive callus (Chap. 5). Similarly, enhanced healing of experimental fractures occurs in the denervated limbs of rats (Aro et al. 1981).

Physical exercise may be necessary for normal growth and could thus be a contributory factor in the retardation of growth in children with chronic diseases (Malina 1969). It might also be involved in the seasonal variation in growth: in the UK, children grow faster in the summer than in the winter months (Marshall 1971).

Malnutrition will interfere with growth and improved nutritional status will restore growth (Graham and Adrianzen 1972).

The lower the social class or socio-economic status of the mother, the smaller the baby and child, but this may reflect the fact that the lower the social class the smaller the parents (Habicht et al. 1974).

During the past 100 to 200 years there has been a profound change in the pace of maturation and to a lesser extent in the ultimate size of individuals in 'developed' countries (Wyshak and Frisch 1982). A century ago the average male did not reach his final height until 23 years. He now reaches it by 17 years. Likewise, the age of the menarche has dropped from 17 to 13 years. The cause of this secular trend is unknown and improved nutrition is unlikely to be the whole answer.

Finally, age has an effect on osteogenesis. Fracture healing is less efficient with increasing age and reduced bone production is thought to be involved in osteoporosis of the elderly.

References

Altner PC, Grana L, Gordon M (1975) An experimental study on the significance of muscle tissue interposition on fracture healing. Clin Orthop 111: 269–273

Anderson HC (1969) Vesicles associated with calcification in the matrix of epiphyseal cartilage. J Cell Biol 41: 59–72

Anderson HC (1976) Matrix vesicle calcification. Fed Proc 35: 105–176

Arey LB (1974) Developmental anatomy. A textbook and laboratory manual of embryology, 7th edn. WB Saunders, Philadelphia London

Aro H, Eerola E, Aho AJ, Penttinen R (1981) Healing of experimental fractures in the denervated limbs of the rat. Clin Orthop 155: 211–217

Ashton BA, Allen TD, Howlett CR, Eaglesom CC, Hattori A, Owen M (1980) Formation of bone and cartilage by marrow stromal cells in diffusion chambers in vivo. Clin Orthop 151: 294–307

Asling CW, Hurley LS (1963) The influence of trace elements on the skeleton. Clin Orthop 27: 213–264

Barzell US, Morecki R, Spigland I (1971) Enchondral (provisional) calcification in vitro. The effect of some metabolic inhibitors. Clin Orthop 78: 191–194

Bassett CAL (1962) Current concepts of bone formation. J Bone Joint Surg [Am] 44: 1217–1244

Bassett CAL, Becker RO (1962) Generation of electric potentials in bone in response to mechanical stress. Science 137: 1063–1064

Bassett CAL, Pawluk RJ, Becker RO (1964) Effects of electric currents on bone in vivo. Nature 204: 652–654

Bassett CAL, Pawluk RJ, Pilla AA (1974) Bone repair by inductively coupled electromagnetic fields. Science 184: 575–577

Baylink D, Wergedal J, Stauffer M (1971) Formation, mineralization and resorption of bone in hypophosphatemic rats. J Clin Invest 50: 2519–2530

Becker RO (1961) The bioelectric factors in amphibian limb regeneration. J Bone Joint Surg [Am] 43: 643–656

Becker RO (1978) Electrical osteogenesis—pro and con. Calcif Tissue Res 26: 93–97

Becker RO (1979) The significance of electrically stimulated osteogenesis: More questions than answers. Clin Orthop 141: 266–274

References

Becker RO, Spadaro JA (1972) Electrical stimulation of partial limb regeneration in mammals. Bull NY Acad Med 48: 627–641
Beighton P (1977) Inherited disorders of the skeleton. Churchill Livingstone, Edinburgh London New York
Bonucci E, Dearden LC (1976) Matrix vesicles in aging cartilage. Fed Proc 35: 163–168
Brown JB, Harrison P, Smith MA (1978) Oestrogen and pregnanediol excretion through childhood, menarche and first ovulation. J Biosoc Sci [Suppl] 5: 43–62
Bulmer MG (1970) The biology of twinning in man. Clarendon Press, Oxford
Buring K (1975) On the origins of cells in heterotopic bone formation. Clin Orthop 110: 293–301
Calhoun NR, Smith JC Jr, Becker KL (1975) The effect of zinc on ectopic bone formation. Oral Surg 39: 698–706
Castle WE (1941) Size inheritance. Am Nat 75: 488–498
Chambers TJ (1978) The cellular basis of bone resorption. Clin Orthop 151: 283–293
Cozen L (1972) Does diabetes delay fracture healing? Clin Orthop 82: 134–140
Crawley RH, McKeown T, Record RG (1955) Parental stature and birth weight. Am J Hum Genet 6: 448–473
Fallon MD, Whyte MP, Teitelbaum SL (1980) Stereospecific inhibition of alkaline phosphatase by L-tetramisole prevents in vitro cartilage calcification. Lab Invest 43: 489–494
Felix R, Fleisch H (1976) Role of matrix vesicles in calcification. Fed Proc 35: 169–171
Fell HB (1956) Skeletal development in tissue culture. In: Bourne GH (ed), The biochemistry and physiology of bone. Academic Press, New York San Francisco London, pp 401–441
Fell HB, Mellanby E (1952) The effect of hypervitaminosis A on embryonic limb bones cultivated in vitro. J Physiol (Lond) 116: 320–349
Fischbein S, Nordqvist T (1978) Profile comparisons of physical growth for monozygotic and dizygotic twin pairs. Ann Hum Biol 4: 417–430
Fishman WH, Ghosh NK (1967) Isoenzymes of human alkaline phosphatase. Adv Clin Chem 10: 255–370
Fleisch H, Russell RGG, Straumann F (1966) Effect of pyrophosphate on hydroxyapatite and its implications in calcium homeostasis. Nature 212: 901–903
Frame B, Jackson CE, Reynolds WA, Umphrey JE (1974) Hypercalcemia and skeletal effects of chronic hypervitaminosis A. Ann Intern Med 80: 44–48
Friedenstein AJ (1968) Induction of bone tissue by transitional epithelium. Clin Orthop 59: 21–35
Friedenstein AJ (1973) Determined and inducible osteogenic precursor cells. In: Hard tissue growth, repair and remineralization. Elsevier, New York, pp 169–181 (Ciba Foundation Symposium II)
Galton F (1889) Natural inheritance. Macmillan, London New York
Graham GG, Adrianzen T (1972) Late 'catch-up' growth after severe infantile malnutrition. Johns Hopkins Med J 131: 204–211
Griffiths GC, Nichols G, Asher JD, Flanagan B (1965) Heparin osteoporosis. JAMA 193: 91–94
Habicht J-P, Martorell R, Yarbrough C, Malina RM, Klein RE (1974) Height and weight standards for preschool children. Lancet I: 611–614
Hall BK (1970) Cellular differentiation in skeletal tissues. Biol Rev 45: 455–484
Hall BK (1978) Developmental and cellular skeletal biology. Academic Press, New York San Francisco London
Hambridge KM, Neldner KH, Walravens PA (1975) Zinc, acrodermatitis enteropathica, and congenital malformations. Lancet I: 577–578
Hamilton WJ, Boyd JD, Mossman HW (1962) Human embryology (prenatal development of form and function), 3rd edn. W Heffer and Sons, Cambridge
Harris WH, Travis DF, Friberg U, Radin E (1964) The *in vivo* inhibition of bone formation by Alizarin Red S. J Bone Joint Surg [Am] 46: 493–508
Harris WH, Lavorgna J, Hamblen DL, Haywood EA (1968) The inhibition of ossification in vivo. Clin Orthop 61: 52–60
Hauspie RC, Das SR, Preece MA, Tanner JM (1982) Degree of resemblance of pattern of growth among sibs in families of West Bengal (India). Ann Hum Biol 9: 171–174
Houston CS (1978) The radiologists' opportunity to teach bone dynamics. J Can Assoc Radiol 29: 232–238
Hurley LS (1981) Trace metals in mammalian development. Johns Hopkins Med J 148: 1–10
Jameson S (1976) Effects of zinc deficiency in human reproduction. Acta Med Scand [Suppl] 593
Jotereau FV, Le Douarin NM (1978) The developmental relationship between osteocytes and osteoclasts. A study using quail–chick nuclear marker in enchondral ossification. Dev Biol 63: 253–265
Kaitila I, Wartiovaara J, Laitinen O, Saxen L (1970) The inhibitory effect of tetracycline on

osteogenesis in organ culture. J Embryol Exp Morphol 23: 185–211
Kim KK (1976) Calcification of matrix vesicles in human aortic valve and aortic media. Fed Proc 35: 156–162
Kiviluoto O (1976) Use of free fat transplants to prevent epidural scar formation. An experimental study. Acta Orthop Scand [Suppl] 164: 1–75
Kochar DM (1977) Cellular basis of congenital limb deformity induced in mice by vitamin A. Birth Defects 13: 111–154
Langenskiöld A, Kiviluoto O (1976) Prevention of epidural scar formation after operations on the lumbar spine by means of free fat transplants. Clin Orthop 115: 92–95
Lindholm TS, Törnkvist H (1981) Inhibitory effect on bone formation and calcification exerted by the anti-inflammatory drug Ibuprofen. Scand J Rheumatol 10: 38–42
Loutit JF, Nisbet NW (1979) Resorption of bone. Lancet II: 26–28
Mack PB, Lachance PA, Vose GP, Vogt FB (1967) Bone demineralization of foot and hand of Gemini–Titan IV, V, and VII astronauts during orbital flight. AJR 100: 503–511
Malina RM (1969) Exercise as an influence upon growth. Review and critique of current concepts. Clin Pediatr 8: 16–26
Marshall WA (1971) Evaluation of growth rate in height over periods of less than one year. Arch Dis Child 46: 414–420
Minaire P, Meunier P, Edouard C, Bernard J, Courpron P, Bourret J (1974) Quantitative histological data on disuse osteoporosis—comparison with biological data. Calcif Tissue Res 17: 57–73
Montgomery WW, van Orman P (1967) The inhibitory effect of adipose tissue on osteogenesis. Ann Otol Rhinol Laryngol 76: 988–997
Moore LA, Huffman CF, Duncan CW (1935) Blindness in cattle associated with constriction of the optic nerve and probably of nutritional origin. J Nutr 9: 533–551
Mosier HD Jr, Jansons RA (1970) Effect of x-irradiation on selected areas of the head of the newborn rat on growth. Radiat Res 43: 92–104
Mosier HD Jr, Grossman HJ, Dingman HF (1965) Physical growth in mental defectives. A study in an institutionalized population. Paediatrics 36: 465–519
Ornoy A, Atkin I, Levy J (1980) Ultrastructural studies on the origin and structure of matrix vesicles in bone of young rats. Acta Anat (Basel) 106: 450–461
Owen CA Jr, Tyle GM, Flock EV, McCall JT (1970) Heparin–ascorbic acid antagonism. Mayo Clin Proc 45: 140–145
Owen M (1970) The origin of bone cells. Int Rev Cytol 28: 213–238
Owen M (1977) Precursors of osteogenic cells. Calcif Tissue Res [Suppl] 24: R19
Owen M (1980) The origin of bone cells in the postnatal organism. Arthritis Rheum 23: 1073–1079
Persson B (1980) Insulin as a growth factor in the fetus. In: Ritzen M, Aperia A, Hall K, Larsson A, Zetterberg A, Zetterstrom R (eds), The biology of normal human growth. Raven Press, New York, pp 213–221
Prockop DJ, Kivirikko KI, Tuderman L, Guzman NA (1979) The biosynthesis of collagen and its disorders. N Engl J Med 301: 13–23, 77–85
Raisz LG, Canalis EM, Dietrich JW, Kream BE, Gworek SC (1978) Hormonal regulation of bone formation. Recent Prog Horm Res 34: 335–356
Rasmussen H (1968) The parathyroids. In: Williams RH (ed), Textbook of endocrinology, 4th edn. WB Saunders, Philadelphia, pp 847–965
Rathbun JC, MacDonald JW, Robinson HMC, Wanklin JM (1961) Hypophosphatasia: A genetic study. Arch Dis Child 36: 540–542
Riekstniece E, Asling CW (1966) Thyroxine augmentation of growth hormone-induced enchondral osteogenesis. Proc Soc Exp Biol Med 123: 258–263
Rimoin DL (1977) Pathogenetic mechanisms of limb malformations in the skeletal dysplasias. Birth Defects 13: 339–353
Riska EB, Michelsson JE (1979) Treatment of para-articular ossification after total hip replacement by excision and use of free fat transplants. Acta Orthop Scand 50: 751–754
Rø J, Sudmann E, Marton PF (1976) Effect of indomethacin on fracture healing in rats. Acta Orthop Scand 47: 588–599
Robinson RA (1979) Bone tissue: Composition and function. Johns Hopkins Med J 145: 10–24
Robison R (1923) The possible significance of hexosephosphoric esters in ossification. Biochem J 17: 286–293
Rosenquist JB, Baylink DJ, Spengler DM (1977) The effect of beta-aminoproprionitrile (BAPN) on bone mineralization. Proc Soc Exp Biol Med 154: 310–313
Sayegh FS, Solomon GC, Davis RW (1974) Ultrastructure of intracellular mineralization in the Deer's antler. Clin Orthop 99: 267–284

References

Schajowicz F, Cabrini RL, Simes RJ, Klein-Szanto AJP (1974) Ultrastructure of chondrosarcoma. Clin Orthop 100: 378–386
Shepard TH (1976) Catalog of teratogenic agents. Johns Hopkins Press, Baltimore London
Short RV (1980) The hormonal control of growth at puberty. In: Lawrence TW (ed), Growth in animals. Butterworth, London, pp 25–45
Siffert RS (1951) The role of alkaline phosphatase in osteogenesis. J Exp Med 93: 415–425
Sinclair D (1978) Human growth after birth, 3rd edn. Oxford University Press, London New York Toronto
Singh S, Padmanabhan R (1979) Effect of chlorpromazine on skeletogenesis. The result of maternal administration of the drug in experimental rats. Acta Orthop Scand 50: 151–159
Smith DW (1977) Growth and its disorders. WB Saunders, Philadelphia Toronto London
Smith DW, Truog W, Rogers JE, Greitzer LJ, Skinner AL, McCann JJ, Harvey MAS (1976) Shifting linear growth during infancy: Illustration of genetic factors in growth from fetal life through infancy. J Pediatr 89: 225–230
Smith R (1979) Biochemical disorders of the skeleton. Butterworth, London Boston
Spadaro JA (1977) Electrically stimulated bone growth in animals and man. Review of the literature. Clin Orthop 122: 325–332
Tanner JM (1972) Human growth hormone. Nature 237: 433–439
Tanner JM, Whitehouse RH, Hughes PCR, Vince FP (1971) Effect of human growth hormone treatment for 1 to 7 years on growth of 100 children, with growth hormone deficiency, low birth weight, inherited smallness, Turner's syndrome and other complaints. Arch Dis Child 46: 745–782
Ten Cate AR, Syrbu S (1974) A relationship between alkaline phosphatase activity and degradation of collagen by the fibroblast. J Anat 117: 351–359
Tonna EA (1966) A study of osteocyte formation and distribution in ageing mice complemented with ^{3}H proline autoradiography. J Gerontol 21: 124–129
Vaughan J (1981) Osteogenesis and haematopoiesis. Lancet II: 133–135
Walton A, Hammond J (1938) The maternal effects on growth and conformation in Shire horse–Shetland pony crosses. Proc R Soc Lond [Biol] 125: 311–335
Weiss P (1950) Perspectives in the field of morphogenesis. Q Rev Biol 25: 177–198
Weston PD, Barrett AJ, Dingle JT (1969) Specific inhibition of cartilage breakdown. Nature 222: 285–287
Winter JSD (1978) Prepubertal and pubertal endocrinology. In: Falkner F, Tanner JM (eds), Human growth. Ballière Tindall, London, pp 183–213
Wood BJ, Robinson GC (1976) Drug induced changes in myositis ossificans progressiva. Pediatr Radiol 5: 40–43
Wyshak G, Frisch RE (1982) Evidence for a secular trend in age of menarche. N Engl J Med 306: 1033–1035
Yasuda I, Noguchi K, Sata T (1955) Dynamic callus and electric callus. J Bone Joint Surg [Am] 37: 1292–1293

9 Conclusions and Clinical Implications

The study of diseases which are characterized by soft tissue ossification has both pathological and physiological importance. Once the pathogenesis in these diseases is understood, this should provide a rational basis for both treatment and prophylaxis—areas which up to now have been generally unsatisfactory. Moreover, insight into the pathogenesis of ectopic ossification will no doubt lead to an understanding of the physiological situation in which the soft tissues do not ossify. This in turn will lead towards the broader goal of an understanding of the regulation of other aspects of normal bone production.

In all of the diseases in which ectopic bone can occur, two important observations are evident to the clinician. First, not all individuals at risk develop ectopic bone, and second, in those who do, the bone has a curious and characteristic distribution. Only a fraction of patients with trauma, hip replacement, abdominal surgery, burns, paralysis, prolonged coma, visceral neoplasms, chronic venous insufficiency or tetanus, produce ectopic bone (Table 9.1). Furthermore, this difference in susceptibility amongst individuals appears to be consistent for that individual. This is exemplified by the extensive studies of DeLee et al. (1976) on hip replacement. Of 295 patients with previous hip surgery (excluding hip replacement), 22 had developed soft tissue ossification. All 22 developed further ectopic bone with subsequent hip replacement. These authors also noted that if one side was affected after hip replacement, there was a 92% chance of ectopic ossification after replacement of the opposite hip as compared

Table 9.1. Prevalence of soft tissue ossification in 'at risk' situations.

Predisposing condition	Approximate prevalence (%)
Elbow dislocation	8
Repeated minor trauma	3
Fracture-dislocation of the hip	15
Hip replacement	20–30
Burns	2–23
Paraplegia	20–30
Hemiplegia	1.2
Prolonged coma	5–27
Chronic venous insufficiency	10
Vertical abdominal incisions	0.3
Colorectal neoplasms	0.4
Hypoparathyroidism	?
Melorheostosis	?

with an overall risk of 14.6% in their series. Similarly, those individuals who develop soft tissue ossification after blunt trauma seem to be at increased risk for ossification at other sites if exposed to future episodes of trauma (Tredget et al. 1977). Few individuals with visceral neoplasms develop ectopic bone, yet Scheidegger (1939) described a patient with ossification in three separate primary neoplasms and this would again suggest an individual propensity to the production of ectopic bone.

The individual variability in susceptibility to soft tissue ossification may be inherited. Evidence to support this hypothesis is incomplete, but there are already several reports in the literature of similarly affected family members. Tama (1966) described two brothers who developed ossification in upper midline abdominal scars. Three of the 24 patients with ossification of the patellar tendon described by Cole (1937) had similarly affected relatives. Evans (1978) noted soft tissue ossification with much the same distribution in twin brothers who sustained burns. Further evidence to support a genetic predisposition to ectopic ossification is provided by fibrodysplasia ossificans progressiva. A patient with this mendelian autosomal dominant disorder has extensive spontaneous ectopic ossification and in addition is unduly susceptible to ossification after trauma.

If the liability to soft tissue ossification in various 'at risk' situations is inherited, then this would represent an example of an ecogenetic condition. In all ecogenetic conditions, some individuals are rendered unduly susceptible to certain environmental agents by virtue of their genetic constitution. In the case of soft tissue ossification, the environmental agents would include trauma (single major or repetitive minor), burns, hip replacement and immobility secondary to neurological conditions.

If genetic variability is involved in the liability to soft tissue ossification in response to certain environmental situations, then it might be possible to identify the 'at risk' individual. These individuals would then be the focus for attempts at prophylaxis. Histocompatibility (HLA) antigens may provide clues in this direction and a number of studies have compared the distribution of these antigens in patients with various types of ectopic ossification with the distribution in normal members of the population. These results are outlined in Table 9.2. The 'normal' population is, however, composed of a mixture of individuals: those who will and those who will not develop ectopic bone when subjected to an 'at risk' environment. Therefore studies ideally ought to compare the distribution of HLA antigens in patients with ectopic bone with the distribution in those without this complication who have been exposed to a similar environmental risk.

There is a clear and well-accepted association of HLA B27 with ankylosing spondylitis and the spondyloarthritis secondary to Reiter syndrome, inflammatory bowel disease or psoriasis. In each of these conditions there is extensive paravertebral ossification and often periosteal formation of new bone at other sites (see p. 87). Shapiro et al. (1976) found an association of HLA B27 with diffuse idiopathic skeletal hyperostosis (DISH) and suggested that this antigen (or its gene) may somehow be involved in the regulation of ossification. A study of the HLA antigens in 22 patients with fibrodysplasia ossificans progressiva did not, however, support this suggestion (Connor 1981). These patients all had extensive ossification, but no increase in any HLA type was found and those individuals with HLA B27 did not have an atypical or unduly severe disease course. Furthermore, this association of DISH with HLA B27 has not been confirmed in more recent, albeit smaller studies (Weiss et al. 1979, Hunter et al. 1980).

Table 9.2. Histocompatibility antigens in soft tissue ossification.

Condition	Finding	Series
Normal population	7% B27	Brewerton et al. (1973)
Normal population	7.6% B18	Minaire et al. (1978)
Arthropathies		
Ankylosing spondylitis	88%–96% B27	Brewerton et al. (1973)
Psoriasis with peripheral arthritis	11% B27	Lambert et al. (1976)
Psoriasis with spondylitis	75% B27	Lambert et al. (1976)
Reiter syndrome	70%–96% B27	Brewerton and James (1975)
Inflammatory bowel disease	7% B27	Morris et al. (1974)
Inflammatory bowel disease with ankylosing spondylitis	75% B27	Morris et al. (1974)
Diffuse idiopathic skeletal hyperostosis	34% B27	Shapiro et al. (1976)
	nad	Perry et al. (1979)
Neurological conditions		
Paraplegia	25.6% B18	Minaire et al. (1978)
Paraplegia	nad	Weiss et al. (1979)
Paraplegia	nad	Hunter et al. (1980)
Paraplegia	20% B27	Larson et al. (1981)
Trauma		
Hip replacement for osteoarthrosis	nad	Mattingly and Mowat (1980)
Other		
Fibrodysplasia ossificans progressiva	nad	Connor (1981)

nad, no association detected.

Similar studies of HLA antigens in patients with ectopic bone after paraplegia have been conflicting but this confusion might, as indicated above, reflect the need for using patients with paraplegia, but without ectopic bone, as a control group. Only two studies have used this approach. Minaire et al. (1978) found B18 in 26% of 43 paraplegics with ectopic bone, but in none of 25 paraplegics without this complication. Larson et al. (1981) only tested for B27 and found this antigen in 5 of 21 paraplegics with ectopic bone but in none of 22 paraplegics who did not have ectopic bone.

Further studies of HLA antigens in patients with ectopic ossification and controls at similar risk but without ossification would seem worthwhile in order to try and define the 'at risk' individual.

The second clinical observation, that ectopic ossification has a restricted and characteristic distribution, is summarized in Table 9.3. Skeletal muscles are involved in most of these conditions but not all skeletal muscles are equal in this respect. Thigh muscles are especially susceptible, as are paraspinal muscles, the muscles of the proximal arm and the masseters. Involvement of the muscles of the distal limbs, face and abdominal wall is uncommon and certain striated muscles never ossify. These muscles with apparent immunity include: the tongue, the extraocular muscles, the upper esophagus, the diaphragm and the sphincter muscles.

Ligaments and tendons are also prone to ossify and again not all sites seem to be equally liable. The paraspinal ligaments and tendons are particularly susceptible,

Conclusions and Clinical Implications

Table 9.3. Distribution of ectopic ossification.

Predisposing condition	Soft tissue sites involved
Blunt trauma	Proximal limb muscles, masseters, patellar tendon, Achilles tendon, anterior longitudinal spinal ligament, knee collateral ligaments
Hip replacement	Proximal thigh muscles
Burns	Muscles around hip, elbow, knee and shoulder
Paraplegia	Proximal thigh muscles
Quadriplegia or prolonged coma	Muscles around hip, elbow, shoulder and knee
Tetanus	Muscles around elbow, shoulder, hip and knee
Certain arthropathies	Paraspinal muscles and ligaments, periosteal sites
Fibrodysplasia ossificans progressiva	Paraspinal muscles and ligaments, proximal limb muscles, masseters

whereas involvement of more peripheral tendons and ligaments is generally less frequent. Except for skin, other soft tissues rarely or never ossify. This characteristic distribution of involvement is revealed most clearly in patients with fibrodysplasia ossificans progressiva (Chap. 4).

The significance of this curious pattern of ectopic bone has been clarified by the elegant animal studies of cell biologists which have identified the inducible osteogenic precursor cells (IOPC). These cells are believed to be of mesenchymal origin. They resemble fibroblasts in morphology and are found in the connective tissue framework of many tissues. Under certain experimental conditions these cells will transform to osteoblasts and produce bone. Their physiological role is unknown but they are prime candidates for the source of osteoblasts at foci of ectopic ossification.

The tissue distribution of IOPC in experimental animals, as revealed by the amount of bone produced in response to the osteogenic stimulus of a given quantity of bone morphogenetic protein, has been shown to be remarkably similar to that of ectopic bone in man. Thus IOPC are most abundant in the connective tissue of skeletal muscles and tendons and occur with diminishing frequency in the connective tissue of dermis, the lung, the gonads and the eye. Spleen, kidney and liver appear to lack IOPC (Gray and Speak 1979, Ashton et al. 1980). It is thus tempting to speculate that man has IOPC with a similar distribution to that found in experimental animals and that the differential susceptibility of skeletal muscles, ligaments and tendons might reflect fine differences in the distribution of these cells.

The time sequence for development of pathological ectopic ossification in man is very similar to that seen for experimentally induced ectopic bone in animals (see p. 108). Further, the scanty sequential histopathological studies on developing ectopic bone in man reveal stages apparently comparable to those seen in experimental animals. This fundamental similarity provides hope that the results derived from the animal models may be applicable to the human situation. If this is the case, then studies with these models should be equally useful in developing our understanding of the physiological function of the IOPC and identifying agents which can prevent their conversion to active osteoblasts.

The reason for the differences amongst species and for the individual variation observed in man in susceptibility to ectopic ossification is not known. It might reflect the concentration of IOPC or be due to quantitative differences in the regulatory mechanisms of these cells. If indeed this variable susceptibility is genetically determined, then presumably the normal ability to prevent ectopic bone formation is under genetic control.

Age also has an effect upon the frequency of ectopic ossification. Fibrodysplasia ossificans progressiva represents the extreme of human susceptibility to ectopic ossification, but even in this condition ossification is episodic with long periods of apparent quiescence. Episodes also have a characteristic age-related frequency. They are infrequent in infancy, increase to a maximum frequency in childhood, decrease in adolescents and become infrequent in later adult life. Similarly, both ossification after muscle trauma and pseudomalignant myositis ossificans are virtually restricted to individuals in their second or third decades. The reason for this age-related change is unknown, but is also seen with induced ectopic bone in experimental animals and so, again, animal studies may shed light on the human situation (Irving et al. 1981).

Experimentally, IOPC can be activated by trauma, contact with certain cell types and demineralized bone matrix (bone morphogenetic protein). In man, ectopic bone can also complicate various forms of trauma as well as occurring in several other, seemingly diverse, conditions (Table 9.1). Limb immobility is a common factor in some of these conditions, but the mechanism by which trauma or immobility activates cells with osteogenic potential in either man or animals is unknown.

Visceral neoplasms can stimulate local mesenchymal cells to produce bone and might do this by direct cellular contact or by production of bone morphogenetic protein. These possibilities could be explored by placing tumor cells from an ossifying neoplasm in a diffusion chamber and implanting it into the muscle of an experimental animal. If the surrounding host connective tissue ossified then a diffusible agent, such as bone morphogenetic protein, rather than direct cellular contact would be favored.

One further mystery in relation to ectopic bone in man is its persistence. In experimental animals IOPC only produce bone as long as an inducing stimulus is present: the ectopic bone is then resorbed. In man, despite the seemingly transient nature of the stimulus in most cases, resorption of ectopic bone is rare except in children who recover from burns or neurological conditions and occasionally with post-traumatic ossification or pseudomalignant myositis ossificans. The mechanism by which trauma or other inciting agents produces persistent ectopic bone must thus involve either some continuing stimulus to bone production or some interference with spontaneous resorption.

In experimental animals certain tissues, for example spleen and kidney, not only lack IOPC but also have an inhibitory effect on the induction of ectopic bone. The mechanism of this effect is unknown: it could be mediated by cellular contact or by local production of a humoral inhibitor. Human adipose tissue also appears to have an inhibitory effect on osteogenesis and, as indicated below, this may have several potential clinical applications (Montgomery and van Orman 1967, Riska and Michelsson 1979). The variation in susceptibility to ectopic ossification amongst individuals and amongst species could be explained by differences in a physiological inhibitory mechanism which prevents activation of IOPC. However, at the present time such an inhibitory mechanism remains speculative.

Despite the lack of understanding of the pathogenesis of ectopic bone, the clinician needs to provide optimal care for his affected patients. Current

Conclusions and Clinical Implications

Table 9.4. Current therapeutic recommendations in ectopic ossification.

Cause of ossification	Treatment
Blunt trauma to limb muscles	Initial rest, then active physiotherapy, occasionally excision when mature, ?fat transplant
Trauma to ligaments	Excision if symptomatic
Hip replacement	Excision with fat transplantation
Tetanus	Excision when mature
Burns	Excision when mature
Ossification of the posterior longitudinal ligament	Decompression for myelopathy
Certain arthropathies	Treatment of primary disease
Neurological conditions	Early physiotherapy, excision of posterior elbow lesions, creation of pseudarthrosis by manipulation for hip lesions or ?excision with fat transplant
Surgical incision	Excision when mature
Chronic venous insufficiency	Excision if recurrent ulceration
Pseudomalignant myositis ossificans	Excision if diagnosis uncertain or there are troublesome symptoms
Ossifying neoplasm	Excision for histology
Fibrodysplasia ossificans progressiva	No known effective therapy

recommendations for therapy in these diseases are summarized in Table 9.4. A few generalizations are possible: patients without symptoms need no treatment; no medication is of proven benefit against established ectopic bone; and the success of excision of ectopic bone depends upon the site, cause and maturity of the ossification. Bone has been successfully excised without recurrence from the posterior aspect of the elbow, surgical incisions and the subcutaneous tissue in chronic venous insufficiency. However, excision of bone from around the hip, regardless of the cause, is almost invariably followed by recurrence. Similarly, excision of bone from the anterior aspect of the elbow is usually followed by recurrence. Patients with fibrodysplasia ossificans progressiva almost invariably have recurrent ossification after excision of ectopic bone from any site.

Before excision of any ectopic bone is considered it is advisable to await maturity of the lesion, as assessed by a stable radiological appearance, normal serum alkaline phosphatase level and decreasing uptake of isotope on serial bone scans. Fat transplantation to the site of excised ectopic bone merits further evaluation as regards sites where recurrence is known to be probable. Effective therapy for fibrodysplasia ossificans progressiva is not yet available, but the animal model suggests that retinoic acid or local injections of somatostatin or antifibronectin may be worthy of clinical investigation (see p. 112). In this and other conditions new therapies should be evaluated by controlled trials or by comparison with the natural history of untreated patients.

Current recommendations for prophylaxis of soft tissue ossification are outlined in Table 9.5 and again reflect the gaps in our understanding of the pathogenesis.

As stressed in Chap. 8, the prevention of soft tissue ossification is only one aspect of the normal regulation of bone production. Ectopic bone is similar, if not identical, in many respects to normal bone. These similarities include: histology,

Table 9.5. Prophylaxis of ectopic ossification in 'at risk' situations.

'At risk' situation	Prophylactic measures
Blunt trauma	np
Hip replacement	np
Burns	Early mobilization
Tetanus	np
Neurological conditions	Early intensive physiotherapy
Certain arthropathies	np
Surgical incisions	np
Chronic venous insufficiency	np
Hypoparathyroidism	np
Melorheostosis	np
Fibrodysplasia ossificans progressiva	Avoid muscle trauma, intramuscular injections, careless venepuncture, lump biopsy and excision of ectopic bone; care with dental procedures

np, none proven.

chemical structure, sequence of collagen types during production, matrix vesicle calcification, handling of radioisotopes, response to drugs, and susceptibility to various diseases such as neoplasia or Paget's disease. The study of ectopic bone might thus provide clues to the overall regulation of osteogenesis.

Production of bone is required for skeletal morphogenesis, growth, remodelling and repair of injury. Regulatory mechanisms which control these processes are doubtless complex, as reflected by the wide variety of agents which can interfere with normal bone production (Chap. 8). Table 9.6 indicates some presumed physiological factors which are involved in skeletal matrix homeostasis, but this list is certainly incomplete. Genes are undoubtedly important in skeletal homeostasis and the rapidly advancing knowledge of the human genome will no doubt shed light on this area (McKusick 1980).

Despite our incomplete understanding of these aspects of bone homeostasis, clinical applications have already been discovered. Restoration of defective growth after replacement of the appropriate hormone is well established (Tanner

Table 9.6. Factors in the physiological regulation of osteogenesis.

Requirement for osteogenesis	Regulatory factors
Skeletal morphogenesis	Genes, ?bone morphogenetic protein
Bone growth	Genes, hormones (growth hormone, thryoxine, sex hormones, ?insulin), trace elements (Mo, Zn), vitamins (A, C), mechanical stress, neural influence, ?phosphate, ? bone morphogenetic protein
Remodelling	Genes, sex hormones, mechanical stress
Repair of injury	Vitamins (A, C), ?neural influence, ?bone morphogenetic protein
Confinement of bone to skeleton	Genes, ?cellular interactions

et al. 1971). Appropriate sex hormones have been used to induce premature epiphyseal closure in patients with excessive growth (Zachmann et al. 1975, 1976).

Bone grafting, to stimulate bone production at sites of non-union, has been practised for many years. Conflicting results of early studies may in part have been due to the treatment of the graft with irradiation, heat or chemicals prior to transplantation, as these agents may neutralize bone morphogenetic activity of the matrix (Jonck and Eriksson 1975). In addition to its role in the stimulation of osteogenesis at sites of non-union, demineralized bone matrix is also of value in craniofacial and other bony reconstruction procedures (Glowacki et al. 1981).

Electrical stimulation of osteogenesis was first used clinically in the nineteenth century (Hartshorne 1841, Garrett 1860). Friedenberg et al. (1971) provided the first modern clinical application of electrical osteogenesis and Spadaro (1977) reviewed the numerous recent uses of this technique. Electrical stimulation of osteogenesis has been successfully applied to the treatment of non-union of fractures at diverse sites and to congenital pseudarthrosis of the tibia (Bassett et al. 1977). Undoubtedly, with future increases in understanding of the mechanisms which regulate ossification, further clinical advances will follow and might lead to effective means of prevention and treatment of skeletal malformations and of defective growth other than that due to hormonal deficiency.

The study of rare diseases can provide important insight into normal physiology. Much of our current knowledge of normal metabolic pathways has arisen because of the clues provided by the inborn errors of metabolism. Similarly, the 'exceptions to the rule' should allow elucidation of normal mechanisms of tissue regulation during morphogenesis, growth and homeostasis. This principle is as sound today as when William Harvey wrote about it more than 300 years ago:

Nature is nowhere accustomed more openly to display her secret mysteries than in cases where she shows traces of her workings apart from the beaten path; nor is there any better way to advance the proper practice of medicine than to give our minds to the discovery of the usual law of Nature by careful investigation of rarer forms of disease.

(Letter to John Vlackveld, 24 April 1657)

References

Ashton BA, Allen TD, Howlett CR, Eaglesom CC, Hattori A, Owen M (1980) Formation of bone and cartilage by marrow stromal cells in diffusion chambers in vivo. Clin Orthop 151: 294–307
Bassett CAL, Pilla AA, Pawluk RJ (1977) A non-operative salvage of surgically-resistant pseudarthrosis and non-unions by pulsing electromagnetic fields. A preliminary report. Clin Orthop 124: 128–143
Brewerton DA, James DCO (1975) The histocompatibility antigen (HLA B27) and disease. Semin Arthritis Rheum 4: 191–207
Brewerton DA, Hart FD, Nicholls A, Caffrey M, James DCO, Sturrock RD (1973) Ankylosing spondylitis and HLA B27. Lancet I: 904–907
Cole JP (1937) A study of Osgood–Schlatter disease. Surg Gynecol Obstet 65: 55–67
Connor JM (1981) A national investigation into the clinical, genetic and pathogenetic aspects of fibrodysplasia ossificans progressiva. MD thesis, University of Liverpool
DeLee JG, Ferrari A, Charnley J (1976) Ectopic bone following low friction arthroplasty of the hip. Clin Orthop 121: 53–59
Evans EB (1978) Musculoskeletal changes complicating burns. In: Epps CH Jr (ed) Complications in orthopaedic surgery. JB Lippincott, Philadelphia Toronto
Friedenberg ZB, Harlow MC, Brighton CT (1971) Healing of nonunion of the medial malleolus by means of direct current—a case report. J Trauma 11: 883–885
Garrett AC (1860) Electrophysiology and electrotherapeutic. Boston

Glowacki J, Kaban LB, Murray JE, Folkman J, Mulliken JB (1981) Application of the biological principle of induced osteogenesis for craniofacial defects. Lancet I: 959–962

Gray DH, Speak KS (1979) The control of bone induction in soft tissues. Clin Orthop 143: 245–250

Hartshorne E (1841) Pseudarthrosis. Am J Med Sci 1: 121–156

Hunter T, Dubo HIC, Hildahl CR, Smith NJ, Schroeder ML (1980) Histocompatibility antigens in patients with spinal cord injury or cerebral damage complicated by heterotopic ossification. Rheumatol Rehabil 19: 97–99

Irving JT, LeBolt SC, Schneider EL (1981) Ectopic bone and ageing. Clin Orthop 154: 249–253

Jonck LM, Eriksson C (1975) Some factors affecting bone formation. A review. S Afr Med J 49: 1747–1753

Lambert JR, Wright V, Rajah SM, Moll JMH (1976) Histocompatibility antigens in psoriatic arthritis. Ann Rheum Dis 35: 526–530

Larson JM, Michalski JP, Collacott EA, Eltorai D, McCombs CC, Madorsky JB (1981) Increased prevalence of HLA B27 in patients with ectopic ossification following traumatic cord injury. Rheumatol Rehabil 20: 193–197

McKusick VA (1980) The anatomy of the human genome. J Hered 71: 370–391

Mattingly PC, Mowat AG (1980) HLA antigens in patients with ectopic ossification after total hip replacement. J Rheumatol 7: 582

Minaire P, Beteul H, Pilonchery G (1978) Système HLA chez les blessés médullaires atteints de para-ostéo-arthropathies neurogènes. Nouv Presse Med 7: 3044

Montgomery WW, van Orman P (1967) The inhibitory effect of adipose tissue on osteogenesis. Ann Otol Rhinol Laryngol 76: 988–997

Morris RI, Metzger AL, Bluestone R, Terasaki DI (1974) HL-A-W27—A useful discriminator in the arthropathies of inflammatory bowel disease. N Engl J Med 290: 1117–1119

Perry JD, Wolf H, Festenstein H, Storey GO (1979) Ankylosing hyperostosis: A study of HLA A, B and C antigens. Ann Rheum Dis 38: 72–73

Riska EB, Michelsson JE (1979) Treatment of para-articular ossification after total hip replacement by excision and use of free fat transplants. Acta Orthop Scand 50: 751–754

Scheidegger S (1939) Heterotope Knochenbildung (Beitrag zur Frage der Metaplasie). Schweiz Z Allg Pathol Bakteriol 2: 153–174

Shapiro RF, Utsinger PD, Wiesner KB, Resnick D, Bryan BL, Castles JJ (1976) The association of HLA B27 with Forestier's disease (vertebral ankylosing hyperostosis). J Rheumatol 3: 4–8

Spadaro JA (1977) Electrically stimulated bone growth in animals and man. Clin Orthop 122: 325–332

Tama L (1966) Heterotopic bone formation in abdominal surgical scars. A report of two cases in brothers. JAMA 197: 219–221

Tanner JM, Whitehouse RH, Hughes PCR, Vince FP (1971) Effect of human growth hormone treatment for 1 to 7 years on growth of 100 children, with growth hormone deficiency, low birth weight, inherited smallness, Turner's syndrome and other complaints. Arch Dis Child 46: 745–782

Tredget T, Godberson CV, Bose B (1977) Myositis ossificans due to hockey injury. Can Med Assoc J 116: 65–66

Weiss S, Grosswasser Z, Ohri A, Mizrahi Y, Orgad S, Efter T, Gazit E (1979) Histocompatibility (HLA) antigens in heterotopic ossification associated with neurological injury. J Rheumatol 6: 88–91

Zachmann M, Ferrandez A, Mürset G, Prader A (1975) Estrogen treatment of excessively tall girls. Helv Paediatr Acta 30: 11–30

Zachmann M, Ferrandez A, Mürset G, Gnehm HE, Prader A (1976) Testosterone treatment of excessively tall boys. J Pediatr 88: 116–123

Subject Index

Abdomen, surgery, incision ossification 93, 94–95
Achilles tendon, ossification 25, 26
Achondrogenesis 125
Achondroplasia 125
Activity, bone growth effects 123, 128
Adenomas, bronchial, ossification 45
Adipose tissue
 osteogenesis inhibition 125
 see also Fat
Age, patient, soft tissue calcification 6
Alizarin red S, osteogenesis effects 127
Alkaline phosphatase see Phosphatase
Alkaptonuria 2, 6
Alopecia, FOP 60
Aminopterin, skeletal malformations 126
Amniotic cells, bone formation and 109
Angiography, in differential diagnosis 13
Ankylosing hyperostosis, spinal 28–29, 89–90
Ankylosing spondylitis
 hip ossification 28–29, 87
 HLA B27 87–88, 133
 ossification 87–88
Ankylosis, in neurological ossification 82
Arsenate, osteogenesis effects 127
Arteries
 idiopathic calcification, infantile 6
 pipe-stem calcification 11
Arthritis, enteropathic 89
 HLA B27 89, 133
Arthropathy
 neurotrophic 89
 ossification after 87–90
 psoriatic 88
Ascariasis 126
Atherosclerosis 2

Bamboo spine 88
Bed rest
 bone growth effects 123
 ossification development 32, 33
 osteoporosis induction 123
Beta-aminoproprionitrile, lathyrism induction 127
Biceps femoris, post-traumatic ossification 19
Bismuth, injection calcification 4, 5

Bladder
 autografts, ossification after 109
 transitional cell carcinoma 45
BMP see Bone morphogenetic protein
Bone
 alcoholic extracts 109, 110
 cellular induction 109–110
 chemical induction 110–112
  see also Osteogenesis
 matrix production 117
 metastatic disease 2
 mineralization 117
  abnormal 121
 osteogenic sarcoma, metastases 46
 remodelling 119
 scans, in differential diagnosis 13
 stress piezoelectric effect 123
 teratogens 126
Bone morphogenetic protein (BMP) 110, 111, 113
Breast, osteosarcomas 44–45
Brooker classification, hip replacement ossification 29, 30
Burns, ossification after 31–33, 132
 early mobilization and 32, 33
Bursitis, calcific 3

Calcification
 amorphous 3, 4
 dystrophic 2, 7
  causes 2
 ectopic 1
 heterotopic 1
 implantation, electroencephalogram electrode sites 4
 intra-articular, causes 10
 metastatic 1
  causes 2
 periarticular 10
 vascular, causes 10
Calcinosis
 circumscripta 3
 idiopathic 10
 idiopathic 2 3
 tumoral 2, 3
  childhood 6

Calcinosis *(continued)*
    presentation 7
    universalis 3
        idiopathic 4
Calcitonin 111
Calcium, intravenous, calcification effects 6
Calcium chloride injection, ossification 108
Carcinoid tumors, bronchial, ossification 45
Cartilage, ossifying, membrane-bound vesicles and 121
Cataracts 98
Cells, bone induction 109–110
Charcot joints 89
'Charley horse' 19
Chlorpromazine, fetal ossification delay 127
Chondrocalcinosis 3
Chondrogenesis, chemical induction 110
Chondroplasia, metaphyseal 125
Chromosomes, abnormalities, fetal growth effects 127
Cleft palate, vitamin A-induced 122
Clinodactyly, in FOP 57, 61
Coal miners, implantation calcification 4
Cobblers, thigh muscle ossification 6
Collagen
    chemical induction 110–111
    types, tissue distribution 110, 111
Coma, prolonged
    ankylosis 83
    ossification 76–77, 78–79, 132
Conjunctiva, calcium deposits 6
Connective tissue, IOPC 97
Copper, deficiency, bone malformation induction 122
Corticosteroids
    in neurological ossification 82
    osteogenesis suppression 111–112, 126
    osteoporosis induction 63, 126
    systemic, ossification development 31
Crohn disease, enteropathic arthritis 89, 133
CRST syndrome 2
Cysts, epidermal 43

De Lange syndrome 58
Deafness, in FOP 60
Dental therapy, in FOP 71
Dentin, demineralized, BMP activity 111
Dermatomyositis
    amorphous calcification, 3, 4
    calcification 2
    childhood 6
    radiology 10, 11
Desmoid, limbal, ossifying 43
Diabetes mellitus
    maternal, baby size and 120
    skeletal hyperostosis and 90
Diagnosis, differential 1–16
    angiography 13
    biopsy 14
    ethnic aspects 6
    familial aspects 6
    history taking 3–6
    laboratory tests 9

occupational and recreational aspects 6
physical examination 6–8
radiology 9–13
Diphosphonates
    in FOP 70–71
    side effects 63
    ossification prophylaxis 31, 82, 83
    see also Disodium etidronate
Diseases, maternal, fetal growth effects 127
DISH 28–29, 133
Disodium etidronate
    in FOP 70–71
    matrix mineralization inhibition 126
    neurological ossification 82, 83
    ossification prophylaxis 31
DNA synthesis, inhibition by tetracycline 126
DOPC *see* Osteogenic precursor cells
Drill bones 6, 23
Drug abuse, maternal, fetal growth effects 127
Drug abusers' elbow 24
Drugs, osteogenetic effects 126–127
Dwarfism, mesomelic 125
Dyschondrosteosis 125
Dysplasia epiphysialis hemimelica 13

Ear, middle, ossification 104
    in FOP 60
Ehlers-Danlos syndrome 2, 6, 7
Elbows, post-traumatic ossification 17, 18
Electricity, osteogenesis and 124, 139
Electroencephalogram, electrode sites, implantation calcification 4
Environment, child growth effects 127, 133
Epidural scars, prevention at laminectomy 125
Epinephrine, injection calcification 4
Epiphyses, multiple dysplasia 125
Epitheliomas, Malherbe 43, 101
Estrogen, bone growth stimulation 120
Exercise, physical bone growth effects 123, 128
Exostoses, FOP 63

Factor VIII deficiency 25
Factor XI deficiency 25
Fat
    autotransplantation, re-ossification prevention 23, 30, 83
    subcutaneous
        calcification, causes 9
        necrosis 6
    see also Adipose tissue
Feet, fungal infections, venous insufficiency and ossification 96
Fetal alcohol syndrome 127
Fetus, growth
    chromosome abnormalities and 127
    maternal disease effects 127
Fibrocellulitis ossificans progressiva 54
Fibrodysplasia ossificans progressiva (FOP) 5, 54–73, 133
    age of onset 58, 136
    biopsy misinterpretation 14
    childhood 6
    clinical features 55–60

Subject Index

coexistent myopathy 65–66
early reports 54
electron microscopy 66–67
etiology 67–69
laboratory studies 65
management 70–71
mutation rate 68
natural history 69
pathology 65–67
patient lifespan 69
prevalence 55
radiology 13
signs and symptoms 8
terminology 54
UK distribution 56, 68
unsuccessful therapies 70
Fibromas, ossification 43
Fibromatosis, congenital 6
Fibromyositis, ossifying, neurogenic 75
Fibronectin, antibodies, osteogenesis induction 112
Fibrosarcoma, amorphous calcification 8
Fibrositis ossificans progressiva 54
Fluorosis, posterior longitudinal ligament effects 92
FOP *see* Fibrodysplasia
Fractures, repair
  cellular inhibition 125
  inhibition by drugs 127
  osteogenesis role 119

Gait disturbance, OPLL 91
Gall bladder, epithelium, bone stimulation 109
Genetic counseling, in FOP 71
Genetic disorders, osteogenesis and 125
Gigantism 119
Growth, longitudinal, genetic control 124
Growth hormone
  deficiency, effects 119
  excess, effects 119
  in longitudinal growth 119
  osteogenesis induction 111

Hemophiliacs, ectopic ossification 25
Hallux rigidus, in FOP 56
Hallux valgus, congenital 8
Hands, post-traumatic ossification 18
Harris' (growth arrest) lines 127
Haversian systems, paraplegic ossification 80
Heberden's nodes 89
Hemangiomas, skeletal muscle, ossification 42–43
Hematomas, ossification 24–25
Hemiplegia, ossification after 76
Hemopoietic stem cells, in ectopic bone 113
Heparin
  osteoporosis induction 112
  vitamin C effects 126
Hip replacement, ossification after 27–31, 132
  Brooker classification 29, 30
  clinical features 29
  individual predisposition 28
  management 30–31

pathogenesis 30
pathology 29–30
prevalence 27–28
primary disease factors 28–29
radiology 29
risk factors 28–29
sex ratio 28
HLA B18
  in neurological ossification 81
  in soft tissue ossification 134
HLA B27
  in ankylosing spondylitis 87–88, 133
  in enteropathic arthritis 89, 133
  in hypoparathyroidism 100
  in neurological ossification 81
  in Reiter syndrome 88, 133
  in skeletal hyperostosis 90, 133
  in soft tissue ossification 133–134
Homocystinuria 2, 6
Hormones, and osteogenesis 119–120, 138–139
Hydantoin, skeletal malformations 126
Hydroxyapatite, paraplegic ossification 80
Hydroxyproline, excretion
  in FOP 65
  in neurological ossification 78
Hypercalcemia
  bone resorption and 121
  metastatic calcification 2
Hyperostosis, skeletal, diffuse idiopathic (DISH) 28–29, 89–90, 133, 138
Hyperparathyroidism 2
Hyperphosphatemia
  idiopathic 2
  metastatic calcification 2, 98, 100
Hyperplasia facialis ossificans progressiva 54
Hyperthyroidism
  adult, osteoporosis induction 120
  childhood, bone growth effects 120
Hypocalcemia 98
Hypogonadism, growth effects 120
Hypoparathyroidism 2
  idiopathic 98
  ossification 98–100
    autosomal inheritance 98
  post-thyroidectomy 98
Hypophosphatasia 125
  abnormal bone mineralization 121
Hypophosphatemia, hereditary 100
Hypothyroidism, congenital, bone growth effects 119–120, 123

Ibuprofen, fracture repair inhibition 127
Incisions, surgical, ossification 93–96, 101
  individual predisposition 95
Indomethacin, fracture repair inhibition 127
Infantrymen, drill bones 6
Infants, full-term, maternal size correlation 123
Injection sites, calcification 2, 3, 4, 108
Insulin
  growth effects 120
  osteogenesis induction 112
Iodine, deficiency, skeletal effects 123
IOPC *see* Osteogenic precursor cells

Kidneys
  failure, metastatic calcification 2
  osteogenesis stimulus lack 112
Klippel-Feil syndrome, radiology 13
Klippel-Trenaunay-Weber syndrome 102

L-Tetramisole (levamisole), alkaline
    phosphatase inhibition 126
Laminectomy, scar prevention, adipose tissue
    effects 125
Laparotomy, incision ossification 93
Lathyrism
  beta-aminoproprionitrile-induced 127
  BMP activity lack 111
Levamisole (L-Tetramisole), alkaline
    phosphatase inhibition 126
Ligaments, post-traumatic ossification 25–27,
    134–135
Limbs
  functional immobility, ossification and 79
  malformation
    drug-induced 126–127
    vitamin A-induced 122
Lipofibromas, ossification 43
Lipomas, ossification 42
Liver, osteogenesis stimulus lack 112
Lumbar transverse processes, bridging 93–94
Lupus erythematosus 2
  radiology 10
  systemic 7

Malherbe calcifying epithelioma 43–44
Malnutrition, growth retardation 128
Manganese, deficiency, bone growth effects 122
Mastectomy, radical, incision ossification 93
Mastication muscles, FOP 60
Melorheostosis, para-articular ossification
    102–103
Menarche, age at 128
Meningitis, tubercular, ossification 76
Menopause
  premature, FOP 60
  venous insufficiency and ossification 96
Menstruation disorders, FOP 60
Mental deficiency, stature and 127
Mesenchyme
  cell derivatives 117, 118
  tissue derivatives 117, 118
Mesenchymomas, ossification 43
Midbrain center, growth influence 127
Middle ear, ossification 104
  in FOP 60
Milk-alkali syndrome 2
Monckeberg medial sclerosis 3
Multiple sclerosis, ossification 76
Münchmeyer's disease 54
Muscles
  skeletal
    calcification, causes 9, 134–135
    hemangiomas 42–43
  strength, bone growth effects 123
Myo-osteosis 17
Myositis fibrosa generalisata 54

Myositis ossificans
  'benign' 22
  circumscipta, idiopathic 5
  neurotica 75
  progressive, localized 103
  pseudomalignant 5, 6, 46–50, 103
    age-related 136
    angiography 13
    clinical features 47
    natural history 48, 50
    pathology 47–48, 49
    radiology 11, 47
    sites 47
    terminology 46–47
  traumatica 5, 17
Myxoliposarcoma, in FOP 69

Nails, dystrophy 98
Neck
  dissection, incision ossification 93
  trauma, ligament ossification 27
Nervous system, disorders, ossification 75–86
Nevi, cutaneous, ossification 43, 101

Obesity
  in skeletal hyperostosis 90
  venous insufficiency and ossification 96
Ollier disease 102
Opiates, injection calcification 4, 24
OPLL see Posterior longitudinal ligament
Osgood-Schlatter disease, patellar tendon
    ossification 25
Ossification
  neurological 75–85
    clinical features 77–79
    history 75
    natural history and management 82–83
    nomenclature 75
    pathogenesis 81
    pathology 80–81
    prevalence 75–77
    radiology 79–80
    spontaneous regression 82
  post-traumatic 5
    experimental 108–109
  soft tissue
    age-related 6
    causes 3, 135
    current therapies 137–138
    local symptoms 5–6
    prevalence 132
    prophylaxis 138
    sites 135
Osteoarthrosis 89
Osteoblasts
  alkaline phosphatase levels 121
  bone matrix production 117
  mesenchymal origin 117, 118
  working lifetime 118
Osteochondrofibrosarcomas 45
Osteoclasts, marrow stem cell origin 118
Osteocytes, alkaline phosphatase levels 121

Osteogenesis
  alkaline phosphatase role 120–121
  cellular interactions 125
  electricity effects 124, 139
  genetic disorders 125, 133–134
  hormones and 119–120, 138–139
  imperfecta 125
    hyperplastic callus 13
  mechanical stress and 123, 124
  medication effects 126–127
  normal 118–119
    requirements 119
  regulation 117–131, 138
  trace element role 122–123
  vitamins and 121–122
Osteogenic cells, origins 117–118
Osteogenic precursor cells
  determined (DOPC) 113–114, 118
  inducible 21–22, 30, 46, 68–69, 81, 97, 112–114, 135–136
Osteogenin 110
Osteoid sarcomas 45
Osteoma cutis, primary 101
Osteomas
  neurogenic 75
  parosteal 38
Osteopetrosis 125
Osteophytes, spinal 89
Osteoporosis
  bed rest-induced 123
  FOP 63, 64
  heparin-induced 126
  hyperthyroidism-induced 120
  neurological ossification 79
  sex hormone deficiency-induced 120
Osteosarcoma
  BMP 111
  bone, radiology 13
  parosteal 38–40
    clinical features 38
    radiology 11
    trabeculation 39
  soft tissue 7, 40–42
    age factors 40
    pathogenesis 41–42
    radiology 11, 40–41

Paget's disease 2
  alkaline phosphatase levels 121
  ectopic bone 26
'Para-ostéoarthropathie' 74
Paraplegia
  connective tissue edema 80
  heterotopic ossification 75
  traumatic, soft tissue ossification 74–86
Parasites, calcification 2, 6
Patellar tendon, ossification 25–26
Pellegrini-Stieda disease 26–27
Penicillamine, collagen conversion block 127
Peritendinitis, calcific 3
Phleboliths 3, 42–43
Phosphatase, alkaline
  inhibition by levamisole 126

levels
  in FOP 66
  in neurological ossification 77–78
  osteogenesis and 120–121
Physiotherapy, in neurological ossification 81, 82
Piezoelectric effect, in bone 123
Pigs, FOP 68
Pilomatrixomas, ossifying 43–44
Pinna, calcification and ossification 7
Pneumonia, in FOP 69
Poliomyelitis, ossification after 76, 77, 78
Posterior longitudinal ligament, ossification (OPLL) 91–92
  ethnic prevalence 91
Prostaglandin E, in FOP 67
Prostatectomy, suprapubic, incision ossification 94–95
Protein
  bone morphogenetic (BMP) 110, 111, 113
  synthesis, inhibition by tetracycline 126
Prussian's disease 23
Pseudohypoparathyroidism 6
  ossification 98–100, 101
Pseudo-pseudohypoparathyroidism, ossification 98–100, 101
Pseudosarcomas, ossification 43
Pseudoxanthoma elasticum 2, 6, 7
Psoriasis, arthropathic 88
Puberty, precocious, growth effects 120
Pyle disease 125

Quadriplegia, ossification after 76, 78
Quinine, injection calcification 4, 24, 109

Rabbit muscles, traumatic ossification 108–109
Radiotherapy, osteosarcoma after 42
Reiter syndrome 88
Retinoic acid see Vitamin A
Rhabdomyolysis 2
Rhabdomyosarcomas, embryonal 43
Rheumatoid arthritis, juvenile, radiology 13
Rickets, vitamin D-resistant 100
Rider's bone 23
Road traffic accidents, ossification after 17
Rothmund syndrome 2

Sacrococcyx, ossifying teratomas 44, 45
Sacroiliac joints, bony ankylosis 88
Sacrotuberous ligament, ossification, in hypoparathyroidism 99
Sarcoidosis 2
Sarcomas
  osteogenic, juxtacortical 38
  synovial 7
Scleroderma 7
  calcification 2
  radiology 10
Scurvy, osteogenesis impairment 122
Seamstresses, ischiogluteal bursae calcification 6
Seborrhea, in FOP 60
Sex hormones

deficiency, osteoporosis induction 120
  growth and 120, 139
Sexual development, FOP effects 60
Skeletal hyperostosis, idiopathic diffuse (DISH) 28–29, 89–90
  HLA B27 133
  terminology 89
Skin
  calcification, causes 9
  ectopic ossification, in hypoparathyroidism 98
  ossifying tumors 43–44, 101
Socio-economic status, stature and 128
Somatomedins, bone collagen synthesis rate 119, 120
Somatostatin, osteogenesis induction 112
Spinal cord
  compression, OPLL 91
  injury, para-articular ossification 75
Spine, cervical
  FOP 60
  longitudinal ligament ossification 27
Spleen, osteogenesis stimulus lack 112
Spondylitis ossificans ligamentosa 28–29, 89–90
Spondylosis hyperostica 28–29, 89–90
Sports injuries, ossification 17
Starvation, in FOP 69
Stature
  correlation coefficient in twins 124
  maturation pace enhancement 128
  mental deficiency and 127
  polygenic inheritance 124
  socio-economic factors 128
Stiff man syndrome 104
Stress piezoelectric effect, in bone 123
Syndesmophytosis 88

Tendons
  calcification, causes 9
  post-traumatic ossification 25–27
Teratoid mixed tumors 45
Teratomas, visceral, ossification 44
Testosterone, bone growth stimulation 120
Tetanus
  ossification after 33–34
  para-articular ossification 34
Tetany 98
Tetracycline, ossification inhibition 126
Thalidomide, skeletal malformations 126
Thigh, blunt injury, ectopic bone 19, 20, 134
Thoracotomy, incision ossification 93
Thrombophlebitis, ectopic ossification 25
Thumbs, short, in FOP 57, 61
Thyrotropin, osteogenesis induction 111
Thyroxine, chondrogenic and osteogenic effects 120
Toes, malformations, in FOP 54, 55–56, 61, 62
Tomography, computerized, in differential diagnosis 13
Trabeculation 2–3, 4
  ectopic ossification and 11, 12
Trace elements, and osteogenesis 122–123
Trauma
  fibrodysplasia ossificans progressiva and 59
  minor, ossification after 23–24
  ossification after 17–37
  clinical features 17–19
  individual predisposition 16
  management 22–23
  natural history 22
  pathogenesis 21–22
  pathology 20–21
  prevalence 17
  radiology 19–20
  terminology 17
  zonal phenomena 20–21
Tumors
  giant cell, ossification 43
  metastatic calcification 2
  osseous, pseudomalignant 41
  ossifying 38–53
    presentation 7
  see also Calcinosis, tumoral and tumor types and sites
Twins
  monozygotic, FOP 68
  stature correlation coefficient 124

Ulcerative colitis, enteropathic arthritis 89, 133
Ultrasound, in differential diagnosis 14
Uterus, constraints, fetal growth effects 123

Venous insufficiency, chronic, ossification 96–98, 101
Vesicles, membrane-bound
  calcification and 121
  osteoblast origin 121
Viscera, tumors
  mesenchyme stimulation 136
  ossification 44–46
Vitamin A
  bone matrix homeostasis 121
  deficiency, bone growth effects 121
  excess
    bone malformations and 122
    bone resorption and 121
  osteogenesis induction 112
Vitamin C
  bone matrix homeostasis 121
  cofactor to hydroxylases 122
  deficiency, osteogenesis impairment 122
  heparin activity inhibition 126
Vitamin D
  bone mineral homeostasis 122
  overdosage, metastatic calcification 2
Vitamin D-resistant rickets 100
Vitamins, osteogenesis role 121–122

Warfarin, skeletal malformations 126
Weight-lifting, ossification after 19
Werner syndrome 2
Wharton's jelly 117

Xeroradiography, in differential diagnosis 9
XYY syndrome 104

Zinc, deficiency, bone maturation effects 122